Other books by Clarence Bass:

RIPPED
The Sensible Way to Achieve Ultimate Muscularity

RIPPED 2
The All-new Companion Volume to *RIPPED*

RIPPED 3
The Recipes, the Routines & the Reasons

THE LEAN ADVANTAGE
Four Years of the Ripped Question and Answer Department

THE LEAN ADVANTAGE 2
The Second Four Years

THE LEAN ADVANTAGE 3
Four More Years

LEAN FOR LIFE
The Lifestyle Approach to Leanness

Challenge Yourself

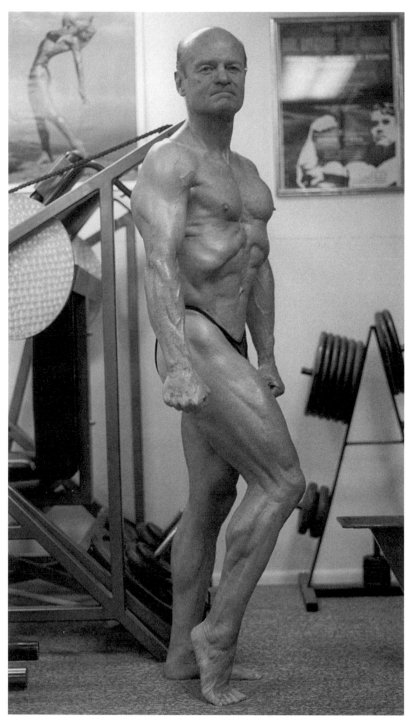

The author at 60. *Photo by Pat Berrett*.

Challenge Yourself

Leanness, Fitness & Health

at any age

by Clarence Bass

Clarence Bass' RIPPED™ Enterprises
Albuquerque, New Mexico

ISBN 0-9609714-7-5

Published by Clarence Bass' Ripped Enterprises
528 Chama, N.E.
Albuquerque, New Mexico 87108 U.S.A.
505-266-5858   FAX 1-505-266-9123
E-mail: cncbass@aol.com
Web Site: http://www.cbass.com

RIPPED is the trademark of Clarence and Carol Bass.

Library of Congress catalog card number: 99-90116

ISBN 0-9609714-7-5

Composition by Wright Graphics
Albuquerque, New Mexico

Manufactured by Thomson-Shore, Inc.
Dexter, Michigan, U.S.A.

Photo on front cover by *Pat Berrett*
Photos on back cover by *Pat Berrett* and *Guy Appelman*

WARNING

Any application of the recommendations set forth in the following pages is at the reader's discretion and sole risk.

The information in this book is intended for people in good
health. If you have medical problems—of any nature—see your
doctor before starting a diet and exercise program. Furthermore,
even if you have no known health problems, it is advisable to
consult your doctor before making any major changes in your
lifestyle.

Invariably, if you are out of shape and want to start training,
follow the advice of the American Medical Association: "Start
slowly and increase the vigor and duration of the activity as
your fitness improves."

To Matt, who in his own way is a musclehead
just like his Dad—and much more.

CONTENTS PAGE

CHAPTER SIX:

CHAPTER SEVEN

PROLOGUE: The Quest Continues

My son, Matt, who lives in another state, recently asked his mother whether I'm having trouble adjusting to getting older. "I can't help wondering," he said, "he's always been so active." Carol thought for a moment and responded, "I've never heard your father obsess or complain about his age." Pausing again, "He just keeps changing, going from one challenging goal to the next."

Secret of Success

That's true. I've never thought of myself as declining with age. To the contrary, I've always seen myself as getting better in one way or another. When I started training at about 13, my goal was self improvement; that's what motivated me. Almost 50 years later, my goal is the same. I believe that's the secret of my success. I don't think of training as a rear guard action, holding off the ravages of age. I never try to maintain; I always strive for gains. There may come a time when I can't find areas in which I can improve, but that's a long way off; it may never come. That's why, at 61, I'm more enthusiastic than ever about training.

I've always said that picking up a barbell is the best thing I ever did for myself. With each passing year, as I continue to train and learn, that becomes increasingly true. As you'll see, weights have always been the bedrock of my training, the one constant. Weight training has been—and is—my ace in the hole, so to speak.

My father, a medical doctor, introduced me to weight training. He brought home a set of weights for his own use when I was a kid. He inspired and encouraged me to train primarily by example; he never pushed me. He was a track-and-field champion during his school-boy days, excelling in the discus, broad jump, high jump, and pole vault. He was practically a one-man team, and I wanted to follow in his footsteps. Mainly, however, I wanted to be "strong." So I started training off and

1

on with my Dad's weights when I was about 12, and by age 13 or 14 I was training regularly. I was on my way.

Crucial First Victories

Like most youngsters, my body responded well to the "iron pills." I had a pretty good physique by the time I was 15. But my first big success, the experience that taught me the satisfaction that comes from working hard and achieving a goal, came in 1954 when I was a junior in high school. I won the New Mexico State High School Pentathlon Championship, a five event contest made up of push-ups, chin-ups, jump reach, bar vault and the 300-yard shuttle run. Weight training, of course, gave me

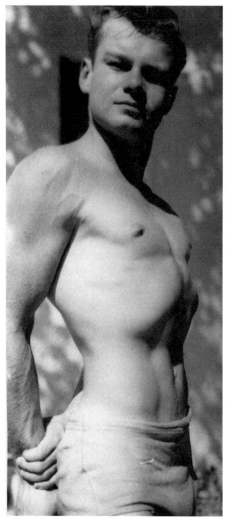

the basic strength to win that first trophy. In particular, I remember that I leapt higher than any other competitor in the jump reach. I know now that the extra spring in my legs came from heavy weight training, something the other boys weren't doing.

About the same time, my father read in our local newspaper that Steve Klisanin had come to Albuquerque to play football at the University of New Mexico. Steve had won the Junior Mr. America title in 1954 and went on to become Mr. America and Mr. Universe in 1955 and 1956, respectively. He was also an accomplished Olympic lifter, rated among the top 10 in the world in the 198-pound class. My father went to the Albuquerque YMCA, where Steve was

I had a pretty good physique by the time I was 15. Photo by my Dad.

doing his weight training, and asked him to come to our home gym and give me a few pointers on the Olympic lifts. I remember how excited I was when Steve showed up at our front door and later commented favorably on my potential in the three Olympic lifts. To make a long story short, with Steve's encouragement—and a lot of hard training—I became one of the youngest lifters in the country to officially Clean & Jerk 300 pounds. I went on to win city, state and regional championships. On the national level, I placed second in the teenage championships two years, second in the YMCA Nationals, and was twice second in the Junior Nationals. My all-time best Olympic lifts were: Military Press 275, Snatch 245 and Clean & Jerk 325.

Law School

During this time I also attended the University of New Mexico law school and, in 1962, graduated second in my class. Some might wonder how I found the time and energy to go to law school when I was obviously devoting substantial effort to lifting. The truth is that weight training made me a better student. Lifting taught me early on that working at something conscientiously pays dividends. The habits I developed in weightlifting—especially consistency—carried over into law school and beyond. Law school, in turn, taught me to think logically, which helped in my training. It was a win-win situation.

Progress Stops

By the time I reached my mid-thirties, however, I realized that further progress in the Olympic lifts would be difficult. So I began to look around for a new goal, something at which I could reasonably expect to succeed. That's when my interest turned to bodybuilding. I was already heavily muscled in the lower back, traps and thighs, the areas most stressed by Olympic lifting. But in the arms, upper back, chest and calves, strong points for bodybuilders, there was plenty of room for improvement. I was also carrying some extra bodyfat, another area where bodybuilders have the edge.

I've always admired bodybuilders. When I was 15, my father and I attended the 1953 Mr. America contest, where we marveled at the physique of winner Bill Pearl. At that time, the national championships in Olympic lifting were held in conjunction with the Mr. America contest every year. My dad and I attended many of these dual championships. We especially enjoyed seeing our friend Steve Klisanin win the Mr. America title in 1955.

3

Inspired by Seipke

Nevertheless, it wasn't until I saw Vic Seipke win the 1976 Past-40 Mr. America contest that I decided to enter bodybuilding competition myself. I had seen Vic win the 1955 Junior Mr. America—I was a senior in high school and competed in the

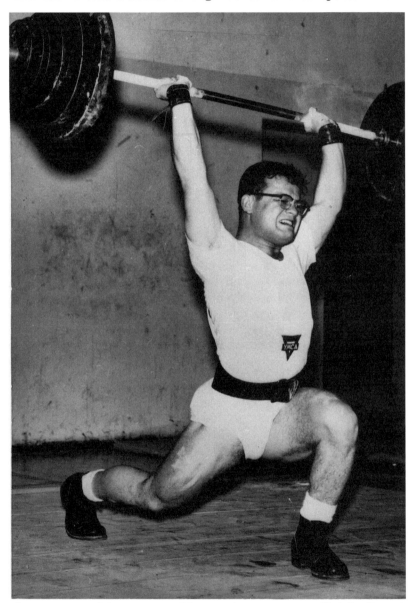

I became one of the youngest lifters in the country to officially Clean & Jerk 300 pounds.

Junior National Olympic Lifting Championships held along with the Jr. Mr. A—and I was one of the judges when Seipke became the first master's national physique champion. I was thrilled to see Vic looking as good in 1976 as he had in 1955. Think of it, more than 20 years had passed and he still looked as great as I remembered! That set my juices flowing again. Inspired by Seipke's success, and realizing my potential, I decided to try to become a master's physique champion myself. And I succeeded.

Another Decade of Improvement

In 1978, I won my class in the Past-40 Mr. America contest, and the next year I won my class again at the Past-40 Mr. U.S.A., along with the overall awards for Best Abdominals, Best Legs and Most Muscular Man. Those victories led me to write *Ripped*, my first book, which explains how I trained for those contests, and in the process reduced my bodyfat to 2.4%.

My success in master's bodybuilding competition motivated me to spend more than a decade improving my physique. The results are recorded in photos throughout the six books that followed *Ripped*. My three-book *Ripped* series, (*Ripped*, *Ripped 2*, and *Ripped 3*) covers all aspects of training for the ultimate physique. My question-and-answer columns in Joe Weider's *Muscle & Fitness*, the world's premier bodybuilding magazine, are collected in *The Lean Advantage 1, 2, & 3*, which are broader in scope, covering fitness, health and fat loss. Finally, *Lean For Life* explains my lifestyle approach to training and focuses equally on weight training and aerobic exercise; it's for the millions of fitness-minded individuals who now seek the benefits of both strength and endurance training.

Most runners and other endurance athletes now supplement their training with weights, while bodybuilders use endurance exercise to help them lose fat and develop aerobic fitness. This connection between strength and endurance athletes led me to an exciting new area for improvement.

Challenge of Rowing

As detailed in *The Lean Advantage 3*, I took up indoor rowing to help me stay lean and found it so challenging that I entered competition. Indoor rowing competition, which simulates rowing on the water using a machine made by the Concept II company, believe it or not, is a lot like Olympic lifting. It requires power in the legs and back, as well as endurance. When I discovered that the rowing motion is similar to the Barbell Clean, where the weight is lifted from the floor to shoulder level in one motion, I

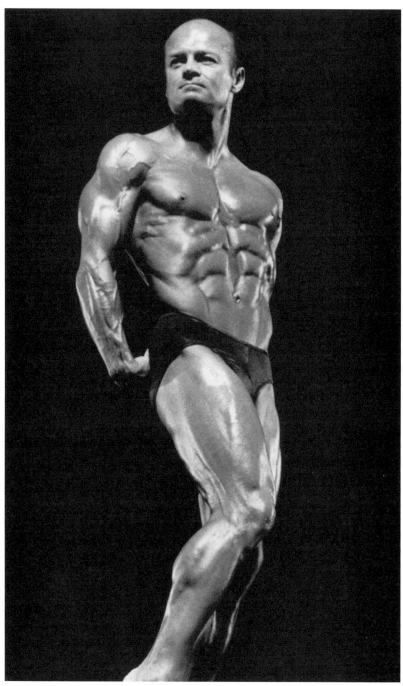

On stage at the 1979 Past-40 Mr. U.S.A., where I won my class and the overall awards for Best Abdominals, Best Legs and Most Muscular Man. *Photo by Ken Sprague.*

was hooked. I entered several competitions and eventually did well enough to rank in the top 25 percent for my age and weight in the 1990 World rankings published by Concept II.

The Cooper Clinic Calls

The next turn in my training career—and still another area for improvement—came about the same time, when Dr. Arno (Arnie) Jensen called from the Cooper Clinic to invite me to come to Dallas for a complete health and fitness evaluation. Arnie said my ideas on diet and exercise, as expressed in my books, were much the same as his. Significantly, he told me that the Cooper Clinic gym now had a fully-equipped weight training area. He also said that I would be the first high-level bodybuilder to be tested at the clinic. That was the beginning of my competition with the treadmill.

As many of you know, Dr. Kenneth Cooper, the founder of the Cooper Clinic, wrote the book *Aerobics*, published in 1968, and was largely responsible for the joggers that flooded the streets across the country and around the world during the '70s. and '80s. So you can see that a call to a bodybuilder from the birthplace of the aerobics movement was a real breakthrough—and challenge.

My test at the Cooper Clinic confirmed Jensen's belief that a combination of weight training and aerobics, balanced training, would produce very positive results. For example, my initial performance on the treadmill put me one and one-half minutes above the 99th percentile for men 50-59 and in the top group for men of any age. Jensen pronounced my overall health "superb."

Treadmill Rematch

I spent the next year doing a variety of endurance exercises, along with my weight training, and returned for a rematch with the Cooper Clinic treadmill in 1989. My training paid off; this time I stayed on the treadmill for 29 minutes, one minute more than before, which put me two and one-half minutes above the 99th percentile for men my age, and in the top category for men under 30.

Three years later, in 1992, when I turned 55, I returned to the Cooper Clinic for another go at the treadmill. My time was 28:38, half way between my earlier tests. I was especially pleased with this result, because I recorded a maximum heart rate of 190 beats per minute. This is significant because the rule of thumb is that maximum heart rate declines one beat per year even for those who continue to train hard. At 55, my predicted maximum heart rate was 165 (220 minus 55 = 165). So, I demonstrated that the expected decline in maximum heart rate as a person ages *can* be substantially altered by training. Chalk up another one for challenge and the total fitness lifestyle.

Last year, when I was 60, I again performed above the 99th percentile on the Cooper Clinic treadmill. Later this year, I plan to challenge myself again with another trip to the Cooper Clinic.

Full Circle

Most recently, my continuing pursuit of improvement has come full circle, back to the lifts that served me so well in my youth. It happened in an unexpected and delightful way.

I couldn't believe my eyes! After not seeing him for almost 40 years, out of the blue my boyhood hero Steve Klisanin appeared at my front door. He was coming through Albuquerque after visiting friends and relatives in the East and decided to look me up. What a pleasure it was to see him again. The memories came flooding back as we got re-acquainted. One of the things we reminisced about was the Olympic lifts.

That delightful conversation with my old friend, combined with a demonstration of the Power Clean I witnessed at New Mexico State University, rekindled my interest in the quick lifts. I started incorporating the Power Clean and the Power Snatch, where the bar is pulled from the floor to arms length overhead in one smooth movement, into my workouts. Happily, after a break-in period, my body has responded well to both exercises, and I'm making good progress. As a matter of fact, I'm now relearning the Squat Snatch, were the bar is caught over head in the full squat position. I'd forgotten how much fun the quick lifts can be—and how much spring they add to the legs. Voila, I've found another area for improvement.

So, Matt—and readers of this book—there's no need to worry about me. With the aid of weight training—and a continuing thirst for improvement—I'm still getting better at 61.

Follow my lead. Turn to chapter one—and challenge yourself.

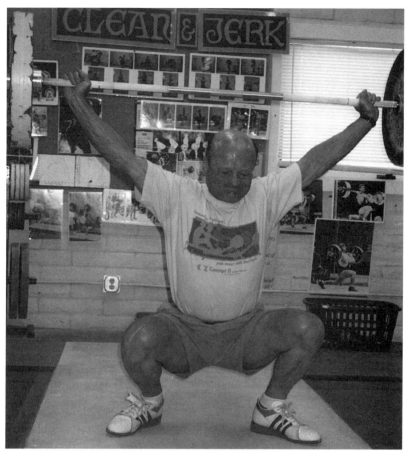

Relearning the Squat Snatch at 60. *Photo by Carl Miller.*

CHAPTER ONE

Challenge Yourself

Challenge Yourself

Always strive to improve. Never be content to rest on your laurels. Making progress toward a challenging goal is what keeps you motivated. Challenge lights the fire. Progress keeps it burning bright. The key is to continually challenge yourself in an intelligent and thoughtful way. That's what this book is about.

A man who had been fat all his life—he weighed 260 pounds when he graduated from high school and gained steadily up to 330 —wrote to me not long ago. With the help of my books, he'd lost 120 pounds, reducing his waist from 49" to 37". He was justifiably proud of himself, but he had a problem. His wife said he should be happy with his vastly improved condition. She complained that he was obsessed, because he wasn't satisfied. He wanted to take additional inches off his waist and harden up more. He was determined to look good at the beach.

After offering congratulations, I told him the fact that he still wanted to improve was a good sign. It was reason to be optimistic that he would not gain the weight back. I sided with him, because in my view working out "to maintain," as many authors suggest, is a sure prescription for failure. "Training is no fun if you're not trying to improve," I told him. "Improvement is what will keep you enthusiastic about eating a sensible diet and training regularly." Finally, I urged him to focus on his own progress and not judge improvement based on other people.

Compete With Yourself

Whether you stay motivated depends to a large extent on how you think about success and failure. Psychologists call this goal orientation. Some people have a competitive orientation; they determine success or failure with reference to other people. Others have an achievement or mastery orientation; they judge success with reference to themselves. They focus on personal mastery and their own improvement. The evidence is strong that people who concentrate on self-improvement—not winning or losing—find it easier to stick with their training.

I've observed this difference time and again; it's almost axiomatic that after every physique contest there will be at least five competitors who think they should have won. They go away feeling like losers because the judges didn't agree. Obviously, they have a competitive goal orientation. I understand their disappointment, but I wish they could see their performance in a more positive light. Only one person can take the top trophy home, but many more go away winners. In my view, the real winner, the person who really benefits from the contest—any contest—is the person who knows he or she did better than ever before, and takes joy in the prospect of making further improvement.

That's what I recommend. Don't allow your motivation to be affected by things beyond your control. Focus on your own progress.

One of the keys to progress is wise goal setting.

Set Specific, Hard Goals

If there is one thing on which motivational psychologists agree, it is that goal-setting is an important source of self-motivation. E.A. Locke's theory of goal-setting is the closest thing there is to a law of nature in the behavioral sciences. According to Locke's theory (published in 1966) specific, hard goals lead to a higher level of motivation and performance than do no goals or a generalized goal of "do your best."

That's why I've long made it a practice to set goals before each training session. It only takes a few minutes with my training diary. During or after every training session I write down my goals for the next time. It's nothing complicated. During weight workouts, I simply note whether I should repeat a movement, add weight or reps, change the exercise, or whatever. After aerobic sessions, I record the workout and jot down ideas on what I should do next.

Make every training session a rewarding experience. Plan your workouts so they produce a feeling of accomplishment. If your workouts are filled with failure, you'll eventually get disgusted

> Psychologists say the cornerstone of motivation is enjoyment. Knowing what makes training enjoyable is the key to staying motivated. Dr. Mihaly Csikszentmihalyi, considered by many to be the world's leading expert on motivation, says enjoyment comes from challenging ourselves with tasks that are neither too difficult or too easy for our abilities.

and quit. On the other hand, if you continually achieve specific, hard goals, you reinforce the training habit. Set yourself up for success. Set goals, but be sure they are realistic. That's very important. Remember: Success breeds success.

The Joy of Striving

Psychologists say the cornerstone of motivation is enjoyment. Knowing what makes training enjoyable is the key to staying motivated. Dr. Mihaly Csikszentmihalyi, considered by many to be the world's leading expert on motivation, says enjoyment comes from challenging ourselves with tasks that are neither too difficult or too easy for our abilities.

It's a subtle point, often missed, that enjoyment comes more from challenge than from achievement. We often think of enjoyment as a "pizza parlor phenomenon." In other words, enjoyment is something that comes after a job is done. Like when teammates celebrate over pizza. We fail to recognize that enjoyment comes mainly from the experience of striving to do a challenging task. The late George Sheehan put it best: "Happiness, we come to discover, comes from the pursuit of happiness."

That means you must keep upping the ante, challenging yourself with new goals. When you get tired of one activity or hit a plateau, move on to a new challenge. As I said, never stop trying to improve. Keep striving—and enjoying. Once you decide to rest on your laurels, you've had it; you're done, you're toast.

A Winning Experience

I've told before how a young woman inspired me to challenge myself more in indoor rowing competition. It's such a wonderful illustration of mastery-oriented, realistic goal-setting that it bears repeating.

In early 1990, I decided to enter an indoor rowing competition at Denver's Cherry Creek Athletic Club. I'd been training on the Concept II rower for several years and decided that competition was just what I needed to push myself to a new personal record for 2500 meters, the standard competition distance at that time.

Importantly, my goal was not to win the competition. That would not have been realistic. I didn't know the other rowers or their rowing times. Frankly, I didn't much care. I had long ago learned that the only competitor that really matters is me. I had no control over the other rowers, but I did know this: If I trained hard, I could probably set a new personal record (PR). For me, that was an appropriate goal—hard, but realistic. In other words, I set myself up for success. It worked beautifully.

I achieved my goal in the qualifying round. I made a new personal record. That made me a winner even though I only placed seventh in the finals. What's more, I got a fix on a challenging new goal.

The personal record I made in the qualifying round was 9 minutes and 47 seconds. It didn't bother me that the winner in my age group did 9:03. The best times are generally by the bigger rowers. He was about six inches taller and outweighed me by at least 50 pounds. It would not have been realistic to judge my success or failure based on his time. But another rower, a young woman, persuaded me that I could do considerably better.

This woman—I later learned she was a collegiate champion on-the-water rower—was about my height and probably weighed a little less than me. Her time was about 9:30, or more than 15 seconds better than my new PR. She rowed with powerful strokes, long and even. She was terrific! Her performance set a bell off in my head. It got me to thinking. She had no height or weight advantage, yet she still beat my time by a substantial margin. That did it. I had a realistic new goal. I knew I could do better—and I did.

In my first rowing session after returning home, I hit a level of performance I would have considered over my head only a few days earlier. With the woman rower as my inspiration, I became convinced that I had sold myself short in Denver. I decided to train for a few weeks at a faster pace, and then go for a new PR. Three weeks later, with my wife Carol as a witness, I made a new PR: 9:32.1.

It was textbook stuff. I set myself up for success by aiming not for a victory, but a new PR. Then, I realistically raised my sights, based on the young woman's performance, and moved on to a new challenge. It was truly a winning experience.

Exercise Advantage Grows

I tell people at every opportunity that exercise and good nutrition become more important with each passing year. People who take care of themselves—challenge themselves—stand out more and more with the passage of time.

"Exercise is one of the real breakthrough areas in the research," says Dr. John Rowe, a recipient of a MacArthur Foundation grant to develop ways to encourage successful aging. "Contrary to received medical opinion until fairly recently," *Fortune* magazine reported, "the case for working out strengthens as we grow older." In support, the magazine cited an eight-year

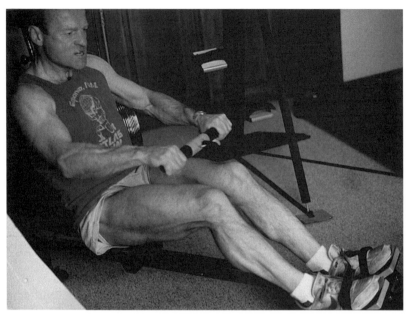

This photo, *taken by my wife Carol*, shows me in the throes of making a new PR, after being inspired by the young woman's terrific performance.

Stanford University study which tracked the health of some 500 runners, ages 50 and over, against a comparable group of non-runners. When the study began, the runners had a 2-1 advantage over the others in various measures of health. At the end, their edge had increased to five times!

"Exercise for young people is an option, but for older people it is an imperative," says Dr. Walter Bortz of Stanford University Medical School and author of *Dare To Be 100* (Simon & Schuster, 1996). Bortz, 60-something and a Boston Marathon competitor, told me recently that he had just purchased a set of weights. Aerobics has many virtues, but Bortz has come to realize that it doesn't fight the fall in bone density and rise in muscle weakness that accompany aging. As documented in *Biomarkers* (Simon & Schuster, 1991), the breakthrough book by William J. Evans, Ph.D. and Irwin H. Rosenberg, M.D., weight training protects and builds the muscle mass and strength which are responsible for the vitality of our whole physiological apparatus.

Lifestyle change can produce dramatic results. A law school classmate of mine was hospitalized with a bleeding ulcer. As soon as he was discharged, he hightailed it to my office to buy a set of my books. From observing me over the years, he said it was obvious I knew something he didn't; he wanted to find out what it was. When I saw him again about six months later, he said he felt like a new man. He looked it, too. He had completely revised his diet and was enthusiastic about his new aerobics and weight training program. Obviously, rather than continue the lifestyle that produced a bleeding ulcer, he decided to adopt the health-and-fitness lifestyle. He decided to challenge himself.

Mental Muscle Responds

In her book, *The Fountain of Age* (Simon & Schuster, 1993), Betty Freidan describes studies by Marian Diamond, an eminent neuroscientist at the University of California at Berkeley, on young and old rats under conditions of varying stimulation.

Instead of standard laboratory conditions (three rats to a small cage), they put some young rats in isolation, in bare, small cages and others in larger cages holding twelve rats, with many objects and mazes to explore. The "enriched rats" were petted and the objects in their cages were changed every week. The researchers found a significant increase in the size of the brains of the young rats in the enriched conditions.

Diamond's group then repeated the experiment with rats from 112 to 142 days (11-14 human years) and 600 days (60 human years). In rats, the brain typically starts to shrivel after 26-41 days, when they become sexually mature. Not only was the shrivelling halted under the stimulating conditions, but actual growth took place in the brains of these rats long after they reached sexual maturity.

> Brain cells do tend to shrink or grow dormant in old age, but that's mainly from lack of stimulation. If we introduce vigorous mental stimulation daily, even an older, developed brain can grow. In short, our mental muscle also responds to challenge.

Finally, hard-to-find geriatric rats were taken out of the bare wire cages in which they had spent their entire lives and put, at 766 days (equivalent to 75 human years), into large cages with stimulating mazes, wheels, blocks and ladders, and other rats. They lived in these cages until 900 days. Believe it or not, these 90-year-old rats showed, again, an increase in both the size and activity of their brain cells. These ancient rats, despite the deterioration that had already taken place, became significantly smarter.

Like any good scientist, Marian Diamond is cautious in the interpretation of her findings. Still, it seems plain enough that brain cells, like muscle tissue, respond and grow when they are used—challenged—even in old age.

In the spring of 1998, Dr. Diamond told *Parade* magazine:

"There is no significant loss of brain cells—in the healthy brains of people who are living normal, healthy lives—all the way up through old age." Brain cells do tend to shrink or grow dormant in old age, but that's mainly from lack of stimulation. If we introduce vigorous mental stimulation daily, even an older, developed brain can grow. In short, our mental muscle also responds to challenge.

The Bottom Line

Take it from Dr. Bortz, Dr. Diamond, me, and many others: Exercise is the best medicine known to humankind. Ignore those who tell you to take it easy. Never stop trying to improve, physically and mentally.

Challenge yourself.

"What [an extremely healthy and creative]
person wants and enjoys is apt to be just what is
good for him!"
                        —*Psychologist Abraham Maslow*

CHAPTER TWO

The Ripped Diet Philosophy Revisited

The Diet Challenge

Diet is a challenge, but not in the usual sense. In my experience, the true challenge of successful dieting is not self-discipline and willpower, but eating satisfaction. The challenge is to both control calories—and be satisfied. Discipline and self-control will bring short-term success. Lasting success, however, comes only with a diet that's filling and satisfying.

Even the word "diet" has a negative connotation. It conjures up thoughts of hunger and deprivation. Diets don't work very well, because they make people unhappy. That's why I never diet. I follow an eating style.

There's no need to eat foods you don't like —I never do—and there's no need to ever leave the table feeling hungry. The secret lies not in how much you eat, but in how and what you eat. If you eat the right foods under the right circumstances, you can eat as much as you want—really want—and still lose fat. It's actually hard to overeat. What happens is you become full and satisfied before you take in more calories than you burn.

Let's start with the circumstances that help you eat only what you really want, and then we'll get to the foods that keep you lean.

Chopra's Rules

In his mind-expanding book *Creating Health* (Houghton Mifflin, 1987) Deepak Chopra, M.D., says, "For most people being fat resides in the mind." Chopra believes the intelligence of our bodies knows what is good for us, and that the first step in bringing one's weight down begins in the mind, starting with an intention to respect the body's intelligence. That sounds nebulous, I know, but you'll see that it makes sense.

Chopra gives some remarkably simple rules to help us activate our inner intelligence:

1. Pay attention to eating.
2. Pause momentarily before eating.

3. Do not sit down to eat if you are upset.
4. Take time to eat, chewing food well and slowly.
5. Stop eating when you are no longer hungry.

As you can see, these guidelines encourage you to observe when you've eaten enough. Chopra explains that the body has a signal for this called the satiety response. He says—this is very important—"It operates quite naturally if the diet has a lot of grains, bulky foods and liquid in it, for these quickly fill you up." Conversely, Chopra adds: "A diet high in fat, salt and sugar tends to throw this response off." Taste enhancers such as these, of course, encourage us to eat more than we really want; they overstimulate our palate.

Nevertheless, "It's not a good idea to fight against strong food cravings," Chopra counsels. They build up and eventually overcome you. He says it's better to try eating half of what you crave, but don't pressure yourself.

Finally, Chopra is convinced that a vegetarian diet is best for health. Still, he wisely points out that including meat and fish in small amounts gives the same health benefits as a strictly vegetarian diet, and is more satisfying.

Like Chopra, I urge people to be flexible. "Backsliding is OK," I wrote in *Ripped 2*. "It takes the pressure off. In fact, an occasional splurge is a good idea." If you really want a pizza, an ice cream sundae or a Big Mac with large fries, you should have it. This frees you up to again pay attention to what your body really wants.

Remember, eating satisfaction is the key.

Calorie Saver Rule #1

Ripped 2 contains a number of techniques I've found useful in helping me control calories and still be satisfied. They're all good, but one stands out above the rest. It has saved me from eating literally thousands of calories I didn't really want. It's so effective that I want you to hear it again.

The only food I put on the table is the food I plan to eat. That's it. I plan my meals and snacks. I know what I'm going to eat. I put everything else away before I sit down to eat.

Leaving food on the table, boarding-house style, is an invitation to overeat. My Dad used to say he never let being full stop him. I'm the same way. Like the comic strip character Hagar, my only limit is that I never eat anything I can't reach.

If extra food is sitting in front of me, I'll probably eat it. If, however, I have to think about it and get up from the table to get more food, I usually won't do it. I realize my true hunger has

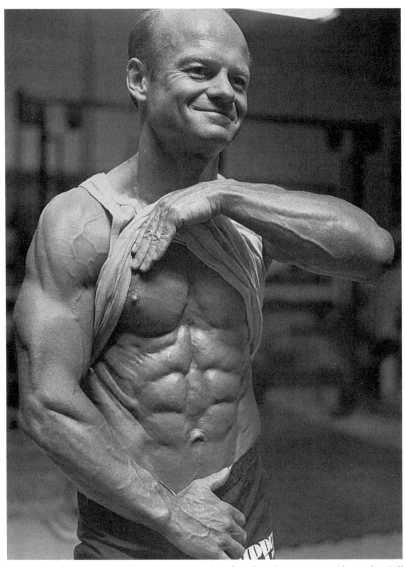

The only food I put on the table is the food I plan to eat. *Photo by Bill Reynolds.*

been satisfied. But if I *really* want more food, I have it, so I won't feel deprived. I know that if I feel dissatisfied at the end of a meal, I'm likely to pick between meals or overeat at the next meal.

Similarly, I don't leave fattening food around the house. It's hard to resist food that stares you in the face every time you go in the kitchen or open the refrigerator. I know that leftovers or sweets present a temptation I usually can't resist. If I see it or smell it, I want to eat it. So I don't bring leftovers home from restaurants or family dinners, and I only eat dessert away from home.

Avoid unnecessary temptation. It works for me. It will work for you as well.

The Core Idea

The core idea of my diet is in *Ripped*, my first book. My subsequent books develop and refine my dietary philosophy. I continue that process in this book. The core idea, however, remains the same: "Avoid concentrated calories."

Sugar and butter are the quintessential examples of concentrated calorie foods. They contain a lot of calories and take up little room in your stomach. They encourage you to overeat. An apple or sweet potato, on the other hand, have a great deal of volume with a low concentration of calories. You can gorge yourself on apples or sweet potatoes and you won't take in more calories than your body can use.

Ripped also imparted a key insight: "By eating only natural, unprocessed foods, you avoid almost all concentrated calorie foods."

I stress whole foods the way they are grown because they provide lots of chewing, tasting and stomach-filling satisfaction, without supplying too many calories. Most foods in their natural form—especially grain, fruit and vegetables—are not fattening. For the most part, it's only when alterations are made—something is added or subtracted—that food becomes fattening.

For those interested in the macro picture, my eating style can be described as high in natural carbohydrates, low in fat (not too low), with plenty of good quality protein for the hardest training athlete. It's balanced—and extremely satisfying.

Finally, I almost never calculate percentages or count calories.

> **New information appears regularly validating the eating style that has kept me lean–and satisfied–for more than 20 years.**

Proof of the Pudding

New information appears regularly validating the eating style that has kept me lean—and satisfied—for more than 20 years. Let's look at a best selling book, an update from the National Institutes of Health, and a recent study.

In *Eating Thin For Life* (Chapters, 1997), her wonderful book about people who have lost weight and kept it off, Anne M. Fletcher, M.S., R.D., calls the eating style I follow "eating large."

Like me, Fletcher's "masters" of weight control focus on the kind of food they eat. Fletcher says that most of them eat "by concept" rather than "by number." For example, only three percent of Fletcher's masters count grams of fat. Many of them told Fletcher they don't know exactly how much fat they eat. (They know it's not a lot.) What they have learned is how to get the most out of their calories. Says Fletcher, "They seek out foods that fill them up but are not fattening." (Sound familiar?)

Fletcher's masters have done the homework necessary to learn which foods are high in fat and calories, and which are not. They know what to eat and what to avoid. One master told Fletcher he goes by two guiding principles: "First, all foods must be low-fat. Second, I eat lots of vegetables and fruits." (Most of Fletcher's masters also eat plenty of whole grains and only a little meat.) This master added another key point: "The simple pleasure of eating natural food in its basic form is great."

To make it "crystal-clear" why eating large works, Fletcher points to an index of food satisfaction developed by researchers from the University of Sidney, Australia. They asked subjects to rate foods according to how full they feel after eating them. Two important concepts emerged.

Calorie for calorie, foods high in fat rate low in satisfaction, and foods low in fat and high in fiber and water (vegetables, fruits and whole grains) were rated more filling. Why? Because, again, low-fat, high-fiber foods take up more room in your stomach. They also take longer to eat, giving the body's satiety response a chance to work.

Secondly, protein-rich foods produce "more satisfying feelings of fullness" than foods high in fat or sugar. "The message," says Anne Fletcher, "is that your meals are likely to stay with you longer if you include small portions of a low-fat protein food," such as chicken, fish, lean beef or non-fat dairy products. (Remember, the Ripped diet has plenty of good quality protein.)

Next, the latest update of the National Institutes of Health conference on "Methods For Voluntary Weight Loss and Control" (*Nutrition*, 12: 672-676, 1996), in effect, endorses the Ripped eating style. "The best means of achieving a healthy weight include adoption of a healthy diet that is low in fat ... and high in fiber ... from whole grains and cereals, fruit, and vegetables," the update states.

The update explains, clearly and concisely, why a diet low in fat and high in natural carbohydrates will put your weight on a downward path: "Because it is easier to eat fewer calories without having to eat small portions."

The eating large concept was also validated in a recent study conducted by Ernst J. Schaefer, M.D. and his colleagues at Tufts University School of Medicine and reported in the *Journal Of The American Medical Association* (1995; 274: 1450-5). These researchers looked at the effect of eating a high-bulk, high-fiber diet containing 15% fat. Importantly, participants were allowed to eat as much as they wanted. As could have been predicted, the subjects lost a significant amount of weight, eight pounds on average.

Why was weight loss predictable? Because the fiber and bulk in the diet took up more room in the stomach. Significantly, the Tuft's study diet weighed 30 percent more than the diet most Americans eat.

The subjects "chose to eat less." As a matter of fact, Dr. Schaefer and his colleagues reported: "Subjects frequently complained about the quantity of food in their diets and of abdominal fullness and satiety."

Clearly, the Ripped diet has stood the test of time.

Now, let's break some new ground.

> The glycemic index (GI) measures the extent to which a given food causes blood glucose, or "blood sugar" to rise. It's really a measure of how rapidly carbohydrates are digested.

The Glycemic Index Conundrum

I wrote about the glycemic index in *The Lean Advantage 2*, but the issue has recently gained new prominence in the war against obesity.

The problem is that some carbohydrates—white bread, instant mashed potatoes, carrots and bananas, for example—are quickly absorbed into the blood stream and may promote the accumulation of fat. The glycemic index (GI) measures the extent to which a given food causes blood glucose, or "blood sugar" to rise. It's really a measure of how rapidly carbohydrates are digested.

On a scale of 0 to 100 (or more), sugar is given a GI score of 100. That's because sugar is pure carbohydrate, very concentrated and rapidly absorbed; it causes a sharp rise in blood sugar. Black beans, on the other hand, score a low 30, because they are slowly digested and cause little increase in blood sugar. Researchers have measured the blood sugar response to hundreds of carbohydrate containing foods and given each a GI rating.

Blood glucose response is important because it triggers the release of insulin. Insulin, in turn, restores blood sugar to normal levels. When a large and rapid rise in blood sugar causes an excessive insulin response, blood sugar drops to below-normal levels. This is called "rebound hypoglycemia" and causes feelings of hunger. It explains why you're hungry again soon after eating sugary foods. But that's not the only concern.

Excess insulin has been called the "supervillain of overweight people" and blamed for the "ballooning of America." That may be a little strong, but an overproduction of insulin caused by eating too many high-glycemic foods is a factor to be reckoned with in controlling body weight.

Insulin is a storage hormone. It acts to store excess blood sugar in the liver and in the muscles in the form of glycogen (sugar for future use). We couldn't survive without insulin to keep our blood sugar in check. As I'm sure you know, abnormally high blood sugar is the hallmark of diabetes, which can cause nerve, eye, kidney and blood vessel damage. The problem is that only a limited amount of glycogen can be stored in the liver and the muscles. What happens to the remaining blood glucose (and the other calories consumed) is why glucose overload, the factor spotlighted by the glycemic index, is a serious issue for people who are overweight.

"Contrary to what many people believe, [blood] sugar is rarely converted to fat," Robert Pritikin (the son of Nathan) explains in *The Pritikin Weight Loss Breakthrough* (Dutton, 1998). Pritikin says most of the blood glucose is quickly burned as fuel. (Remember, high blood sugar is dangerous.) But that doesn't solve the problem, says Pritikin, because the normal energy mix is 50 percent sugar and 50 percent fat. If more sugar is burned for energy, that means less fat is burned. The end result, of course, is that the fat which would have been burned—from stored fat or an incoming meal—accumulates in your tissues. In short, glucose overload encourages fat storage.

That's why the glycemic index is important for people trying to lose body fat.

Unfortunately, predicting G.I. scores can be tricky. We've long known that simple carbs, such as those found in candy, desserts and other sugary foods, are fattening. Simple carbs, of course, carry very high GI scores; sugar, you'll remember, is at the top of the heap with a GI score of 100%. But it was once thought that complex carbohydrates, such as those found in starch-based foods, were not a problem. Now, however, actual testing shows that the effect of starches on blood sugar is quite variable. For example, carrots, a complex carbohydrate food, and honey, a simple sugar, are both in the 80-90% range, while cherries score a low 22% on the glycemic index.

All is not lost, however. There is a logical way to make your way through the glycemic index conundrum. Actually, there are several solutions which can be used separately or in combination. I use them all to varying degrees. Let's take them one at a time.

The Protein Solution

Barry Sears, Ph.D., author of *The Zone* (Harper Collins, 1995), suggests that eating more protein (and less carbohydrate) helps insure that more of the calories you eat are burned for energy, rather than stored as fat. The reason, he says, is the action of "insulin's biological opposite," glucagon.

Insulin makes sure that blood sugar doesn't go too high, and glucagon makes sure it doesn't go too low. As you'll recall, insulin is a storage hormone. It stores excess calories as glycogen or body fat. Glucagon has the opposite effect; it's a mobilizing hormone. Glucagon takes stored glycogen and fat and sends it back into the blood stream to be utilized for energy. Glucagon release is stimulated by dietary protein.

According to Sears, the ratio of carbohydrate and protein in each meal or snack determines whether the calories you eat are stored as fat or mobilized for energy. He suggests that by eating 40 percent carbohydrates and 30 percent protein, along with 30 percent fat, you increase glucagon and lower insulin.

But Dr. Bob Arnot, in his *Revolutionary Weight Control Program* (Little, Brown, 1997), cites research that a 20 percent protein diet cuts blood glucose—and therefore insulin response—significantly.

The Ripped diet is in between those two figures, at about 25 percent protein. I include some good quality protein in every meal or snack, but I don't worry about the precise ratio of carbs to protein. You'll see that strategy at work in the sample menu plans in the next chapter.

In addition to promoting the release of glucagon, the protein in every part of my diet slows the absorption of carbs, which in turn stabilizes my blood sugar. That keeps me satisfied and feeling good, without overshooting my calorie needs.

Now, let's look at another way to keep blood sugar—and fat accumulation—under control.

Add a Little "Good Fat"

Louis J. Aronne, M.D., author of *Weigh Less, Live Longer* (Wiley, 1996), suggests that people having difficulty losing weight because of blood sugar and insulin problems consider eating a diet that has "slightly higher protein and fat content." We just discussed protein, so let's talk about the role of dietary fat in combating glucose overload. (We'll cover the health benefits of "good fats" in a later chapter.)

It's well known that fat takes longer to digest than carbohydrate or protein; it remains in the stomach longer. *The Univer-*

sity of California At Berkeley Wellness Encyclopedia of Food and Nutrition (Rebus, 1992) says, "Fats...promote a sensation of feeling full when eaten, probably because they slow the emptying of food from the stomach." Fat makes you feel satisfied longer because it causes the food you eat—including carbohydrates—to be released into the blood stream more slowly. That keeps your blood sugar on an even keel, and discourages overeating.

You don't want to overdo a good thing, however. Dr. Aronne suggests eating only "slightly" more fat. Remember that a gram of fat contains more than twice as many calories as a gram of protein or carbohydrate (9 calories to 4). Eating too much fat still makes you fat. Plus, as Robert Pritikin points out, high-fat foods stimulate the appetite. But *a little fat* in the diet can actually help you burn more of the calories you eat, rather than store them in your fat cells.

Some fats do a better job of this than others, however. Foods high in saturated fat (butter, cream, egg yolks, red meat, chocolate, lard and margarine, for example) "make your muscles far more resistant to the effects of insulin, allowing your blood sugar to rise, which increases your glucose load," says Dr. Bob Arnot. Dr. Aronne agrees, but adds that "consuming monounsaturated fats, such as olive or canola oil, may have a tempering effect" on insulin resistance. Personally, I've found that adding a teaspoon of canola oil or a tablespoon of ground flax seeds to meals and snacks makes me feel satisfied longer, and doesn't encourage overeating. Hopefully, they help me burn more—and store less—of the calories I eat as well.

In addition, I frequently add fatty fish such as salmon or sardines to my evening meal. (You'll see this in the sample meal plans.) Fatty fish reduces my risk of having a heart attack or stroke (more about that later), and new research suggests that it may also play a role in keeping me lean.

Japanese researchers investigated the effect of fats on leanness. They raised mice prone to diabetes and obesity on a variety of high-fat (60%) diets, and then measured the change in body weight (*Metabolism*, Vol. 115, No. 12 (December), 1996: pp.1539-1546). Interestingly, body weight gains varied widely depending on the type of fat consumed. For example, mice fed soybean oil or lard gained far more than those fed fish oil.

The discrepancies were truly startling. According to Artemis P. Simopoulos, M.D., author of *The Omega Plan* (Harper Collins, 1998), the difference in weight between the mice fed a soybean-oil diet and those fed a fish-oil diet was "comparable to the difference in weight between a 225- and a 150-pound man." The lard/fish oil comparison produced a weight gain disparity almost as great, according to Dr. Simopoulos. Significantly, all of the diets contained the same number of calories.

The researchers warn that humans may respond differently, but you can see why I'm enthusiastic about adding small portions of fatty fish to my diet on a regular basis.

Finally, let's consider the effect of bulk and fiber on blood sugar levels and weight gain. They may offer the best solution of all to the glycemic index puzzle.

The Whole Food Connection

"By eating only natural, unprocessed foods...you'll become lean," I wrote in *Ripped*. That simple prescription also takes much of the worry out of the glycemic index.

It's really no surprise that instant rice and white bread have GI scores right up there with glucose tablets and jelly beans. Why not? Because they are very refined products, with practically all of the bulk and fiber removed or broken down. White bread is made with highly refined bleached flour, and instant rice has been milled and polished to removed the bran and germ, and what's left has been precooked and then dehydrated. The same is basically true of corn flakes or white bagels. These fractured foods, like simple carbs, quickly break down into glucose, and then mainline into the blood stream, shooting your blood sugar sky high.

But what about bananas and carrots? They are rapidly absorbed and cause a rise in blood sugar even though they are whole foods. Yes, but when you put a banana in your mouth no chewing is required, because the peel has been removed. You just mash the banana and swallow. And carrots have been cooked until they are soft, breaking down the tough cellular walls found in raw carrots. My guess is that raw carrots—I don't know this for sure—do not trigger a major insulin response.

No, I'm not suggesting you eat the banana peel along with the banana or that you abstain from cooked carrots. (Cooked carrots are so low in calories, only 48 in 3.5 ounces, they never made anyone fat.) I'm simply urging you to think about the form of the food you eat. Is it "as grown" or highly processed? Is it hard or soft? If, like a whole apple or broccoli, it requires some heavy duty chewing—takes a while

> **Here's the bottom line on the glycemic index: Include some protein or a little "good fat" with every meal or snack—and stick mainly to unrefined, whole foods. Do that and you can stop worrying about the glycemic index.**

to eat—it's likely to have a low-glycemic effect. On the other hand, if there's no crunch to a food and it goes down in a flash, like apple juice or instant mashed potatoes, your blood sugar is in for a roller coaster ride.

You don't even have to avoid high GI foods. Just remember to mix them with low GI foods. If you want a banana, have it with non-fat, plain yogurt or a few nuts. Mix low-GI beans with rice or potatoes and have cauliflower or zucchini with cooked carrots. These combinations are only moderately glycemic and do not cause havoc with your blood sugar. Plus, they are generally low in total calories.

If you really need to shed body fat, however, it's best to emphasize foods in their very unrefined form. That means eating plenty of whole grains, raw or lightly cooked vegetables and fresh fruits. Eat foods in a form as close as reasonably possible to "as grown."

Take it from me and Dr. Bob Arnot: "It isn't possible to eat as many carbs if they're not refined." Plus, the natural bulk and fiber in whole foods blunt the uptake of carbohydrates and decrease the insulin response.

Here's the bottom line on the glycemic index: Include some protein or a little "good fat" with every meal or snack—and stick mainly to unrefined, whole foods. Do that and you can stop worrying about the glycemic index.

Protein Requirements for Athletes

Finally, no discussion of diet in the bodybuilding field would be complete without touching on protein requirements for athletes. I've consistently said that getting enough protein is not a problem—especially if you consume some good quality animal protein with every meal or snack.

> **Pound for pound, bodybuilders and endurance athletes such as runners actually need about the same amount of protein, but for different reasons.**

Bodybuilders do not need massive quantities of protein. But the old view that exercise doesn't change the need for dietary protein is also wrong. Well-controlled studies demonstrate that hard-training athletes may actually need twice as much protein as an inactive person.

"There isn't an exact number for athletes," registered nutritionist Nancy Clark explained recently in *The Physician and Sportsmedicine*, "because protein needs vary depending on whether an athlete is growing, rapidly building new muscle, doing endurance exercise, or dieting." Significantly, if you work hard at both strength and endurance training or if you're dieting, your protein needs may be the greatest of all athletes.

Protein, from the Greek word meaning "of prime importance," is needed to make red blood cells, produce hormones, boost the immune system, and help keep hair, fingernails and skin healthy. We all need protein because it provides the basic building blocks for repair and maintenance of the body. Protein is especially important for athletes, because it's essential for building muscle and repairing the muscle damage that occurs during training.

Nitrogen balance testing, which measures the protein entering and leaving the body, shows that the U.S. Recommended Daily Allowance for protein—0.4 grams per pound of bodyweight—is adequate for sedentary adults. Athletes, as we said, have special needs and require more protein.

Interestingly, it turns out that, pound for pound, bodybuilders and endurance athletes such as runners actually need about the same amount of protein, but for different reasons. (A 200-pound bodybuilder, of course, requires more total grams of protein than a 150-pound marathoner.)

According to Mark A. Tarnopolsky, Ph.D., one of the most active researchers on the protein needs of active people, endurance exercise increases amino acid oxidation, while resistance exercise speeds protein turnover and muscle protein synthesis. Endurance athletes use protein for energy, especially during intense exercise. That, of course, means they need additional protein for normal repair purposes. Resistance exercise doesn't burn amino acids for fuel but, not surprisingly given that weight training promotes muscle breakdown and growth, it does increase the amount of protein needed for muscle replacement and growth.

According to Dr. Tarnopolsky and Nancy Clark, recent research shows that both strength and endurance athletes need in the range of 0.5 to 0.9 grams of protein per pound each day. The lower end of the range is for recreational exercisers and the top end for elite bodybuilders and endurance athletes in hard training.

Importantly, athletes engaged in sports involving both strength and endurance (e.g. football, wrestling), and dieting athletes have the greatest needs of all; they require up to 1.0 gram of protein per pound of bodyweight.

It's easy to see why. People doing both strength and endurance training—including bodybuilders, like me, who alternate high-intensity weights and aerobics—are burning amino acids during aerobic sessions and, in addition, increasing protein turnover and synthesis in weight training. Dieting athletes, accord-

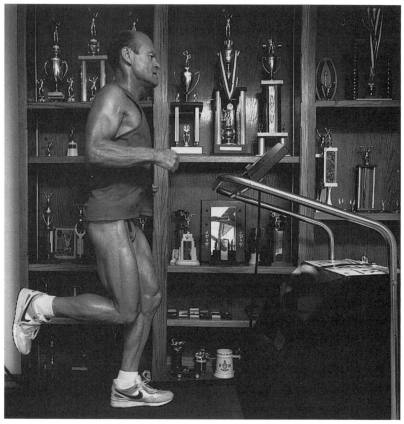

People doing both strength and endurance training—including body-builders, like me, who alternate weights and high-intensity aerobics—may have the highest protein needs of all athletes. *Photo by Guy Appelman.*

ing to Nancy Clark, use protein as a source of energy, particularly when carbohydrates are not available.

Does gender make a difference? Dr. Tarnopolsky says that female endurance athletes require about 25% less protein than men. That's because a woman has more fat and less muscle than a man. Female bodybuilders probably need slightly more protein, however, because they have proportionately more muscle than most other female athletes.

What about vegetarians? Nancy Clark says athletes who choose a vegetarian diet can get adequate protein, but they must be careful to eat a variety of plant foods that have complementary amino acids. For example, a mixture of grains and legumes (rice and beans) contains all essential amino acids. Tofu is also an excellent addition to a vegetarian diet. Says Clark: "Tofu has made headlines because it is a high quality plant protein that contains all essential amino acids and offers the bonus of phytochemicals that protect against heart disease and cancer."

I am a near-vegetarian, and I never count grams of protein. Still, I get plenty of protein, because I make it a practice to include some animal protein with every meal or snack.

Computer analysis by the Cooper Clinic in Dallas shows that my diet easily meets the newly discovered protein requirements for athletes. Based on my training diary—also the source of the sample menus to follow—I consume about 175 grams of protein each day. That's slightly more than one gram per pound, the top amount required by elite athletes doing both strength and endurance training. (The total breakdown of my diet was found to be 26% protein, 55% complex carbs, 18% fat and 1% sugar.)

> I don't like to foster the notion that muscle comes from a bottle. In my experience, intelligent training and a healthy balanced diet are far more important than any of the so called ergogenic aids.

Finally, remember my words from *Ripped 2*: "Excess calories from any source [carbohydrates, fat or protein] build fat, not muscle." There's no need to force down massive quantities of protein.

(You'll find information on protein requirements in all my books, but I'm especially proud of the complete discussion of muscle-building nutrition in *Ripped 2*.)

Creatine

I don't like to foster the notion that muscle comes from a bottle. In my experience, intelligent training and a healthy balanced diet are far more important than any of the so-called ergogenic aids. Teenagers, in particular, should be taught that the surest path to any goal—including meaningful success in sports—involves sustained personal effort.

Nevertheless, creatine monohydrate has become so pervasive that it can't be ignored. It has moved from the pages of bodybuilding magazines, to *Sports Illustrated*, to the front pages of local newspapers. Sales for 1998 were nearly $200 million. There's no getting around the fact that it works for most people. What's more, according to *The Physician and Sportsmedicine*, "no clear evidence of harmful side effects...has yet emerged."

Creatine is an amino acid stored in the muscles. During intense exercise, it facilitates the regeneration of ATP, the chemical that fuels muscular contractions. When more creatine is present, an athlete can work out harder and longer and recover faster. Extra creatine also increases muscle mass, probably from fluid retention inside the muscle cells and/or as a response to harder training.

The normal daily requirement for creatine is about 2 grams for a 150-pound male; about half usually comes from meat or fish in the diet, and the other half is made by the body. A half-pound of raw meat contains about 1 gram of creatine.

Natural levels can be boosted through creatine supplementation. Not surprisingly, vegetarians respond especially well to taking creatine. On the other hand, heavy meat eaters may show little or no effect. The fact that I am a near-vegetarian probably explains my response to creatine.

My first inkling how well creatine works came on one of New Mexico's wonderful hiking trails—after only five days on the supplement. Tres Pistoles Trail is one of our favorites. It's a strenuous hike with a glorious view at the top. What I like best about Tres Pistoles is the relentless nature of the climb. The trail gains elevation from almost the first step; it starts gradually and ends with a heart-pounding segment. I've tested my strength and endurance on this trail numerous times and remember being pleased to reach the top in under one hour the previous year, 59 minutes and nine seconds, according to my training diary.

Well, this time I made it in 51:26.37, a new PR by more than seven minutes. "A really good climb!" I wrote in my diary. I didn't mention creatine—I guess I was still a doubting Thomas—but I remember thinking later, after the effects of the supplement were undeniable—I'd gotten stronger and gained muscle—that creatine helped me motor up that trail in high gear.

My results are apparently not at all atypical. Richard B. Kreider, Ph.D., Associate Professor at the University of Memphis, told *The Physician and Sportsmedicine* that 80% of creatine studies have reported an ergogenic effect. On the basis of research reports and his own observations, Kreider says gains in lean mass and strength are impressive, and occur very fast. Maximum effects, however, occur in about six weeks, and then you're on your own again.

What about side effects? I've had two minor problems—stomach discomfort and muscle cramping—which are relatively common. Others have apparently experienced nausea and diarrhea, both caused by overdosing. Muscle soreness may be another side effect.

I've noticed more muscle soreness after weight workouts since I began taking creatine. At first, I simply ignored the added soreness. I didn't consider it a problem, because it's not unusual for me to be sore after weight workouts. I consider soreness a good thing; it's part of the adaptation process that leads to greater strength once the muscles recover. I always make it a point not to train again while soreness persists; not training again until the soreness is gone insures complete recovery. It also alleviates any possibility of permanent damage to muscle fibers. Plus, there was no mention of soreness in the literature on creatine.

Now, however, at least one study, reported in the *Canadian Journal of Applied Physiology* (23(5): 471, 1998), has found a strong correlation between soreness and creatine supplementation. The researchers didn't attempt to explain how creatine might cause soreness. Perhaps creatine-packed muscle cells are more prone to injury, or it could be that the harder training creatine makes possible produces more soreness. Whatever the connection may be, I consider the additional soreness a minor inconvenience, especially in view of the fact that soreness is generally a result of overload and part of the adaptation process. (We'll discuss the significance of overload in the chapter on training.) Nevertheless, soreness is a factor to be considered when deciding whether to take or continue taking creatine.

The other two problems were easily remedied. I cured the stomach discomfort by switching to "100% pharmaceutical grade creatine," which is a very fine powder and less irritating to the digestive system. (I use a private label brand from a local health food store, but any brand marked "pharmaceutical grade" or a similar designation should be fine.)

> You wouldn't keep pumping gas after your tank is full, and there's nothing to be gained by taking more creatine than necessary to keep your muscles fully loaded.

The cramps I was having in my calves disappeared when I reduced the dosage—to $1/2$ teaspoon, or 2.5 grams, on rest days and 1 teaspoon on workout days, $1/2$ tsp before and $1/2$ tsp after workouts.

That's less than usually recommended on the label. It shows taking the lowest effective dose is the best policy. Your muscles can only hold so much creatine. Taking a maintenance dose is like topping off your gas tank. You wouldn't keep pumping gas after your tank is full, and there's nothing to be gained by taking more creatine than necessary to keep your muscles fully loaded. The amount required, of course, varies with your exercise level and muscle mass. If you weigh 225 and train six days a week, you'll probably need more creatine than a 150-pound person who exercises 2 or 3 times a week.

Finally, it's wise to remember that widespread creatine supplementation is only a few years old. The effects of long-term usage have not been studied.

Obviously, we've still got a lot to learn, but so far so good. Jeff S. Volek, M.S., R.D., a doctoral student in sports medicine at Penn State who will soon launch a long-term study, believes that long-term side effects are unlikely for healthy people. "[Creatine is] a low-molecular-weight compound that is excreted in the kidney by simple diffusion," he told *The Physician and Sportsmedicine*. "In the maintenance phase, people take the amount of creatine generally found in the diet."

"I think creatine is here to stay," Volek added. "It works and people can actually see and feel results."

CHAPTER THREE

New Model Meals

Good Meals Get Better

I feel like a bodybuilder going back into the gym after having made PRs across the board in my last workout. It's daunting. How am I going to top my last performance?

In *Ripped 3*, I explained, meal by meal, eating to become lean the sensible, no-hunger way. I did detailed preparation instructions—and extensive commentary—for 22 meals and numerous snacks, all filling and satisfying but not fattening.

> Until recently, I thought my diet was just about perfect. Nevertheless, I tried to keep an open mind, and I continued to challenge myself. It paid off! My diet evolved—and got even better.

Following up in *Lean For Life*, I thoroughly examined why a low-fat, natural-carbohydrate, near-vegetarian diet will make and keep you lean—and I gave more meal plans. How can I top that?

Frankly, I didn't think I could. Until recently, I thought my diet was just about perfect. Nevertheless, I tried to keep an open mind, and I continued to challenge myself. It paid off! My diet evolved—and got even better.

The model meals presented here incorporate the improvements; they are taken directly from my training diary. Most of the new elements were introduced in the last chapter. Here we'll put them into practice and explain more about why they work so well.

Before we begin, let's go over a few basics to help those who haven't read my other books and refresh the memory of those who have.

No Calorie Count

The model meals do not included a calorie count. There are several reasons for this. First, like the masters of weight control discussed in the last chapter, I eat by concept, rather than by number. Calorie counting or portion control doesn't work, because it's contrary to human nature; denial simply makes us want more. I focus on eating foods that fill me up without giving me too many calories. If you stick to the type of foods included here—and only put on the table the food you plan to eat—the satiety response described by Dr. Chopra will keep your calorie needs and your appetite in balance. You'll feel satisfied naturally. You won't want more.

Rather than count calories, I keep track of how much I eat by following a uniform eating pattern. I eat three main meals and two or three snacks every day—I never miss a meal—and I eat what's described here most of the time. I sometimes deviate on the weekends, but even then, I eat about the same amount. The consistent pattern makes it easy to adjust—add or subtract—as necessary to achieve my goals.

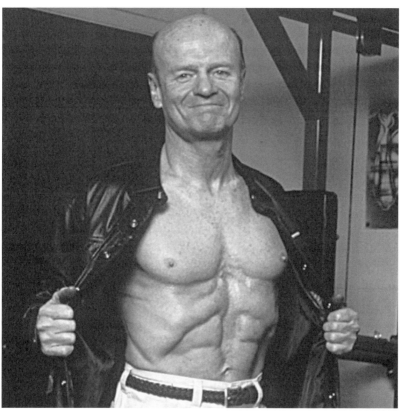

This photo was taken shortly after my 60th birthday, just before I began writing this book. It shows how well the new model meals work. *Photo by Pat Berrett.*

I weigh myself at least once a week—always on the same day and under the same circumstances—to see if I'm gaining, losing or maintaining. I keep a weekly record right by the scale, which makes it easy to see at a glance what has happened to my weight over the last several months.

For many years, I weighed myself on a regular hospital scale and measured my waist with a tape measure—changes in the waistline usually reflect a gain or loss in body fat—but I now use the electrical impedance scale made by Tanita. The Tanita Body Fat Monitor/Scale is the most convenient and accurate device I've found for monitoring weight and body fat at home.

You program it with your gender, height, and whether you're an athlete; it stores personal data for up to four people. Then, you simply tap a button to select your data and step on the scale. In a few seconds, your weight and body fat percentage appear.

Importantly, it's very consistent. Step on the scale 10 times— place your bare feet squarely on the foot pads—and you get the same result almost every time. (See *The Lean Advantage 3* for tips on how to make the best use of body fat test results.)

One rap against the Tanita scale is that the electrical current may not go effectively through the upper body, because the electrodes are only under the two feet. Critics maintain that may skew the accuracy of the body fat reading for people who have a marked difference in upper and lower body fat distribution. That may be true, but I don't believe it's a major concern, because the body's response to diet and exercise is more important than absolute accuracy. The critical factor is whether the measuring device shows progress or lack thereof. In my experience, the Tanita scale does that well.

If you're an athlete, be sure to purchase one of the models with the "athlete" mode; they're specially calibrated for people who exercise regularly and are already relatively lean. Tanita suggests these models for people with a resting heart rate of less than 60 beats per minute, but that's only a rule of thumb. Tanita also says their scales are not recommended for professional athletes and bodybuilders, but I'm very pleased with mine. Tanita scales are widely available and reasonable priced; check with your local sporting goods store or call 1-800-9-TANITA. (By the way, I have no connection whatsoever with Tanita.)

Once you know what's happening to your body weight—and fat—it's relatively easy to add, subtract or substitute food items to get your body moving in the desired direction.

Don't rush the process, however. Make small adjustments, and give them time to work. Generally, it's not a good idea to try to lose more than one pound a week.

As I said in *Ripped 3*: "If you're impatient and try to lose faster, you defeat yourself in three ways: 1) Your metabolism slows down to save energy; 2) You lose muscle tissue; and 3) You get hungry and binge."

It's best to eat *slightly* less and exercise *slightly* more. To increase your activity level, try walking. That's what I do.

If you find it necessary to add more food, do that slowly as well. Keep in mind that muscle is for the most part trained on, not eaten on. Extra calories from any source—carbs, protein or fat—almost always turn up on your body as fat. I never consciously add calories to my diet, even though I'm always trying to gain muscle.

As you would expect, since they are taken from my training diary, the portions in the model meals are what I normally eat. You'll probably require more food or less, depending on your size, body composition and activity level. To give you a basis for comparison, I'm very lean, quite active, and I usually weigh between 155 and 160.

The amount of food you can eat without gaining fat is strongly influenced by how lean you are. That's because muscle is active tissue and burns calories around the clock; fat is inactive and burns few calories. Women, who naturally have less muscle and more fat than men, should keep this in mind when setting up their initial meal plans. Pound for pound, women usually require smaller portions than men. But again, it's a mistake to severely restrict food intake, for a man or a women.

Okay, enough preliminaries, let's get to the new model meals.

My "New" Old Reliable

1 cup (cooked) mixed whole grains (kamut, oat groats and amaranth)
1 cup skimmed milk (0% fat)
3 tablespoons black beans
100 grams (3.5 oz) frozen sliced peaches
1 chopped apple
1 tablespoon flax seeds (ground)
1/2 teaspoon sesame seeds
2 tablespoons protein powder

Earlier versions of this breakfast cereal are in *Ripped 3* and *Lean For Life*. The major changes are the addition of black beans and flax seeds. These new ingredients have a nutritional impact, but the most important thing they add is eating pleasure and long-term satisfaction. Before we get to that, however, let's deal with the nuts and bolts of making my favorite breakfast.

For many years, I've built my breakfast around whole grains.

Oat groats, which are simple hulled whole oats, were included in my earlier books; there's no change here. Kamut and amaranth are the new additions. All three grains are available in most health food stores, and some supermarkets. We buy ours at Wild Oats, the fast growing health food supermarket chain. If there's not a food store like this where you live, my guess is there soon will be.

The new grains are major upgrades discovered by my wife, Carol. Kamut is an ancient form of wheat which flourished in Egypt more than 5,000 years ago. It's easy to see why it is making a comeback in modern times. (A few seeds reportedly recovered from a burial crypt made their way to America after World War II.) It has a delicious taste and texture. But what I like best is its size; it's almost three times as big as regular wheat. You can really get your teeth into it; I love the chewiness.

Amaranth, on the other hand, is one of the tiniest grains. Also an ancient grain—it's touted as the miracle grain of the Aztecs because of the quality protein it contains—amaranth is crunchy and slightly porridgy at the same time. When cooked it becomes gelatinous and makes the entire grain mixture stick together. I like that. Amaranth usually comes in a smaller package than the other grains and you may want to use proportionally less of it.

Oats, kamut and amaranth are currently my favorite combination, but any whole grain or combination of whole grains is fine. They all have about the same number of calories. Other whole grains that I enjoy are rye, wheat and barley.

Whatever grains you select, just add water and cook until done. Most recipes suggest 1 cup grain to 2 cups water, but I prefer a 1 to 3 ratio; the extra water adds bulk to the final product and cuts down on the calorie content.

Grain can be cooked in a big pot on the stove, but it's much easier to use a large automatic rice or grain cooker. With our automatic cooker you simply pour in the grains, add water and turn it on; when the grain is done, the cooker turn itself off. Let it stand until all the water is absorbed and then store in the refrigerator. That's all there is to it. Your part, setting up and putting things away afterwards, takes about five minutes. Make up a week's supply at a time, and it's only a little more trouble to prepare than corn flakes.

I use canned black beans, but you can buy dry beans and cook your own if you have the time. Any kind of beans would work (pinto beans, black-eyes peas, kidney beans, lima beans, navy beans, lentils, for example), but black beans, which are a staple throughout much of Latin America, are my favorite. I believe you can find them in most supermarkets.

Yes, I know that beans may sound like a strange addition to a breakfast cereal, but trust me, you'll like the almost buttery chewiness they add. (More about beans in the comments section.)

We buy frozen peach slices in five-pound bags at our local supermarket; they are frozen at the peak of freshness and have no sugar added. I sometimes substitute a frozen combination mixture (peaches, cantaloupe, honeydew melon, red seedless grapes) which is also available in five-pound bags. Any frozen fruit is fine; just make sure there's no sugar added. Again, if you have time, buy fresh fruit and prepare your own. I do take the time to cut up a fresh apple, because I like the added crunchiness. But the convenience of frozen peaches (and other fruits) is just too much for me to pass up.

Flax seeds are also available in health food stores and most regular supermarkets. You'll need a coffee grinder to grind them into a digestible meal. Like the beans, ground flax seeds add a delightful body—the ground meal absorbs water, forming a mucilage—and crunch that you're guaranteed to like. Again, we'll get to the nutritional benefits momentarily.

To actually put this huge cereal together, start with a cup of cooked grain. Add one tablespoon of protein powder— I use our own milk and egg brand, but any good tasting protein without added fat is fine—and the beans. Stir and pour in the non-fat milk. (If milk doesn't agree with you, try low-fat soy milk; it's not only delicious, but high in good quality protein as well.) Add the frozen fruit and pop the whole mixture into the microwave for about 6 minutes. While the oven is thawing the fruit and taking the chill out of the grains and milk, use the time to chop the apple and grind the flax seed. Take

This breakfast mixture really captures the core idea of the Ripped diet. Made up almost entirely of natural, unprocessed foods, it avoids concentrated calories and provides lots of chewing, tasting and stomach-filling satisfaction.

the heated mixture out of the microwave, stir in the flax seed meal, add the chopped apple and top with another tablespoon of protein powder. (Naturally, we believe our protein is best, and I know there's nothing else on the market that tastes better.) Enjoy.

By the way, you'll need a huge bowl. I use a serving bowl that holds over a quart.

Comment

This breakfast mixture really captures the core idea of the Ripped diet. Made up almost entirely of natural, unprocessed foods, it avoids concentrated calories and provides lots of chewing, tasting and stomach-filling satisfaction.

Cooked whole grains are a perfect example of the foods that have a great deal of volume with a low concentration of calories. As Robert Pritikin writes in *Breakthrough*, "Foods that contain water or are cooked in water… provide fewer calories bite for bite than processed foods that contain concentrated calories." What better example could there be than whole grains which absorb three times their volume in water; remember, I use three cups of water for every cup of grain. Amazingly, when you lift the cooker cover after an hour or so there's no water in sight, only cooked grains.

> **Earlier versions of this breakfast mixture contained practically no fat. This time, however, to slow the absorption of carbohydrates and keep blood sugar on a more even keel, we added a little good fat in the form of flax and sesame seeds.**

Like the cooked grains, the peach slices and the chopped apple are whole foods containing plenty of water and few calories. They're more examples of the type of food you can gorge on without taking in more calories than your body can use.

Earlier versions of this breakfast mixture contained practically no fat. This time, however, to slow the absorption of carbohydrates and keep blood sugar on a more even keel, we added a little good fat in the form of flax and sesame seeds.

Flax seeds are relatively new to the tables of U.S. homes—Carol brought them into our household—but they have been part of the human diet for at least 10,000 years. Mahatma Gandhi once observed: "Wherever flax seeds become a regular food item among the people, there will be better health."

Flax seeds are rich in Omega 3 essential fatty acids and fiber, and low in saturated fat and calories. One tablespoonful of flax seeds, the amount in this recipe, contains only 47 calories, but has a big effect. The fat and the fiber—flax seeds also contain protein—blunt the absorption of carbohydrates. What's more, the freshly ground flax absorbs five times its weight in water. The result is a sticky, thick mucilage, which provides plenty of eating satisfaction. The water, of course, reduces the calories in every bite.

There's only one problem. Flax seeds are so high in Omega-3 fat that one can develop an Omega-6 essential fatty acid deficiency by using only flax seeds over a long period of time. We solve that problem by adding one half teaspoon of sesame seeds, which are a rich source of Omega-6 fats. A shortage of Omega-6 is ordinarily not a concern—the normal American diet is loaded with Omega-6 fatty acids—but on an otherwise low fat diet like mine, adding a few sesame seeds seems like a good precautionary measure. Plus, sesame seeds add a little more fat to slow digestion, and they taste good. (As you'll see, I use sunflower seeds for the same purpose at lunch and in some snacks.)

Beans are not only the best plant source of protein—on average, beans contain about 22 percent protein by dry weight—they are relatively low in calories, virtually fat-free and second only to wheat bran as the best source of dietary fiber. Listen to the UC Berkeley *Wellness Encyclopedia*: "Because [they] are digested slowly, [beans] cause a gentle rise in blood sugar. As a result [those] who eat a substantial amount of beans require less insulin to control their blood sugar." Sounds like just what we're looking for, doesn't it?

The complete protein in this meal is provided by non-fat milk and protein powder. (Like all plant foods, the protein in beans and seeds is incomplete; the one exception is soybeans.) Milk and protein powder were included in the earlier recipes, so that's not a change. As mentioned earlier, I've long made it a practice to include some high quality animal protein in every meal.

Stick to meals like this breakfast, which provide maximum fullness with minimum calories, and you'll become lean and stay lean. Just as important, you'll never be hungry or feel dissatisfied.

My "New" Favorite Lunch

Boca Burger Sandwich:
    2 slices whole grain bread
    1 Vegan Original Boca Burger (fat free)
    1 tablespoon fat-free mayonnaise
    1 teaspoon mustard
    Alfalfa sprouts or lettuce

Cherry Yogurt Mix:
    1 cup plain nonfat yogurt
    1 cup (140 grams) frozen cherries (no sugar added)
    1 tablespoon flax seeds (ground)
    $1/2$ teaspoon sunflower seeds
    1 package Equal (optional)

Those who have read my earlier books will no doubt be shocked—shocked!—to learn that I no longer have a peanut (or almond) butter sandwich every day for lunch. (I still have nut butter occasionally, however.) After all, I became famous for getting ripped, and staying ripped, while eating high-fat nut butter almost every day—for going on 20 years. I'll explain in the next section why peanut butter actually helped me stay lean—and why I changed—but first let's talk about making this lunch.

My current favorite bread is Ezekiel 4:9 Sprouted Grain Bread made by Food For Life Baking Company of Covina, California. According to the wrapper, the recipe is inspired by the Holy Scripture verse: "Take unto thee wheat, and barley, and beans, and lentils, and millet, and spelt, and put them in one vessel and make bread of it... ." Sounds good, doesn't it?

This bread is high in fiber, has no added fat or shortening—and it's wonderfully chewy. Food For Life also makes a bread called Bran For Life which Carol and I like. It has the same number of calories, 80 per slice, and even more fiber, six grams versus three for Ezekiel, but it doesn't have quite as much body or chewiness. We get both breads at Wild Oats, and we've seen them at our regular supermarket from time to time. Look around. I'm sure you can find Food For Life bread or something similar.

The key is to select a whole grain bread, low in sugar and high in fiber. By all means, avoid breads made with refined flour; they have no fiber to speak of and require little or no chewing. They melt in your mouth. You'll find them in the center aisles of supermarkets everywhere. Those are the high-glycemic index breads that drive up blood sugar and encourage fat accumulation. Experiment and find a good chewy bread—read the label—that you really enjoy. Don't try to ferret out the bread with the lowest calorie count. In the long run, eating satisfaction is more important than a few extra calories.

Carol and I discovered meatless Boca Burgers—they're made with soy—by reading Dr. Bob Arnot's *Revolutionary Weight Control Program* (Little, Brown, 1997). Arnot says Boca Burgers can be found at supermarkets across the country. We buy ours at Wild Oats and our regular supermarket. Like Dr. Bob says, they have "a true burgerlike mouth feel and taste." We've tried other veggie burgers. These not only taste good and stay with you, they're very low in fat, relatively low in sodium (high in potassium), yet high in protein and fiber. (More about the nutritional benefits of soybeans shortly.)

Boca Burgers come in three flavors: Vegan Original contains no fat; Hint Of Fresh Garlic is 99% fat free; and Chef Max's Favorite is 98% fat free. We prefer the no-fat version, but you should try them all.

I toast the bread, heat the prebaked, frozen patty in the microwave, spread a little fat free mayo (I use Kraft, 10 calories per tbs.) and mustard (deli mustard with horseradish—and only 10 calories—is my favorite), throw in a big handful of alfalfa sprouts (for added thickness and crunch) and eat. It's quick and easy. (Some people are concerned about bacteria lurking in sprouts. If you're in that group, use lettuce or some other leafy vegetable.)

As an alternative, I frequently substitute chicken for the Boca Burger. Carol buys preboned chicken breasts and freezes 2-ounce portions in individual plastic sandwich bags. I simply put the chicken into the microwave for one minute, turn it over and cook for another minute. Usually that does it, but if any part of the chicken looks like it's not completely done, I cook it more. Then I cut the chicken into small pieces and put it on the bread, along with the mayo, mustard and sprouts or lettuce.

I know two ounces of chicken doesn't sound like much, but I guarantee that it makes a thick sandwich that you can really get your teeth into. That's one of the reasons I switched to a Boca Burger or chicken sandwich for lunch; they require more chewing and take longer to eat than a peanut butter sandwich. That's true even though I always cut the nut butter sandwich into pieces to make it last longer.

This may sound like a trivial point, but it's not. Gulping down your food is a bad mistake. It encourages overeating. Your appetite control mechanism (Dr. Chopra, remember?) doesn't have time to signal your brain when you've had enough. Eat slowly. Take time to savor your food. That way, you'll be far less likely to overeat. (As I said before, I still eat a nut butter sandwich from time to time. The only change is that I now use raw nut butter, rather than roasted, to preserve the integrity of the essential fats.)

Cherry yogurt mix is an upgrade of the mixture I described in *Lean For Life*. Nonfat yogurt, of course, is no change; it has been a staple of my diet for more than a decade. In *Ripped 3*, I explained that I switched from whole milk yogurt to reduce calories—and because I found a brand of nonfat yogurt (Alta-Dena) at our health food store that I really liked.

Other people must have found fat-free plain yogurt to their liking as well, because our regular supermarket now stocks several brands; Dannon and Mountain High are two that I use regularly. Be sure to check the label. If the calorie content is higher than 110 or so, it probably contains some things you don't really want. "Low fat" yogurt, of course, contains fat, and flavored yogurt usually contains more calories. I prefer to add my own sweetener and flavoring.

Don't be afraid to make your meals taste good. Keep in mind that it's important to eat things you really enjoy. That way you'll be happy to stick to the style of eating that will make and keep you lean.

The frozen cherries are new since my last book. Supermarkets now have all kinds of frozen fruit, with no sugar added. Cherries are my favorite, but I also use frozen strawberries, blueberries and, of course, the peaches included in my breakfast recipe. They are all low in calories; the cup (140g) of frozen cherries in this meal contains only 60 calories.

The ground flax seeds and the sunflower seeds are wonderful additions as well. The benefits of including these are the same as explained in connection with my breakfast. The flax and sunflower seeds add a nice crunch and mouth feel.

I usually add a packet of Equal (aspartame) for added sweetness—remember there's no sugar added to the yogurt or cherries—but that's up to you. Don't be afraid to make your meals taste good. Keep in mind that it's important to eat things you really enjoy. That way you'll be happy to stick to the style of eating that will make and keep you lean. Just be sure to put everything away—before you sit down to eat. Don't tempt yourself to eat more than you plan.

A preparation tip: You'll need an oversized cup to hold this mixture. I use a Campbell's soup cup that holds two full cups of liquid. I thaw the frozen cherries (in the big cup) in the microwave for two or three minutes and use the time to grind the flax seeds. I don't grind the sunflower seeds, because I want to retain the crunch of the whole seeds. Take the cherries out of the microwave, add the yogurt, and mix in the flax seed meal and the sunflower seeds.

I eat the yogurt mixture along with the sandwich but you may prefer to have it separately.

This is a good lunch. It's tasty and satisfying without containing too many calories. The cherry yogurt mix is really delicious. I believe you'll enjoy it as much as I do.

Comment

I promised to explain why I didn't—and don't—get fat eating peanut butter. I've already hinted at the reason. Eating satisfaction is critical, if you plan to stick to your diet and stay permanently lean. As I said in *Ripped 3*, I enjoy peanut butter. It's important not to deny yourself foods you like. If you do, cravings start to build and before you know it, you're bingeing. But if you allow yourself a measured amount of foods you like—I never gorge on peanut butter or other fattening foods—you'll always be satisfied, in control—and lean. It's counter productive to purge your diet completely of foods you really like—even when you're tying hard to lose weight.

You've probably guessed part of the reason why I switched

from nut butter to a Boca Burger or chicken sandwich. Here's the whole story. I already explained that a burger or chicken sandwich requires more chewing and takes longer to eat than peanut butter. Peanut butter is a concentrated calorie food; it has lots of calories in a small volume. Chicken and Boca Burger have more volume and fewer calories. A no-fat Boca Burger contains only 84 calories, compared to 172 in two tablespoons of peanut butter; two ounces of chicken breast has about 50 calories. I simply decided I enjoyed lower-calorie chicken or Boca Burger as much or more than peanut butter. Obviously, it was time to switch. (Again, I still eat nut butter sandwiches occasionally; raw almond butter is my current favorite.)

Another reason, of course, was that I wanted to take advantage of the additional protein—a Boca Burger contains 12 grams of protein compared to less than eight in the peanut butter—to promote release of the mobilizing hormone glucagon. As explained in the last chapter, glucagon has the opposite effect of insulin. It shifts metabolism into burning mode, so that the carbohydrate and fat stored in your body is released into the blood stream to be utilized for energy.

Both protein and fat slow the emptying of food from the stomach, so the switch from high-fat peanut butter to high-protein Boca Burger or chicken may be a wash in terms of blood sugar stabilization. That's not clear, however, because soybeans score an extremely low 15 on the glycemic index. Dr. Bob Arnot says, "Soybeans set the record for slow-burning foods." But peanuts, because of their high-fat content, also score very low. Barry Sears places soybeans and peanuts side-by-side at the bottom of his list of foods having a glycemic index of 30 percent or less. Again, it's six of one and a half dozen of the other.

A new protein-quality scale, which is directly applicable to humans, rates soy a perfect 1.0. That's the same as milk and eggs, and slightly better than beef!

One area where soybeans clearly outscore peanuts is protein quality. That's not a surprise, because it's long been known that soy protein contains all of the essential amino acids. A recent development, however, is that a new protein-quality scale, which is directly applicable to humans, rates soy a perfect 1.0. That's the same as milk and eggs, and slightly better than beef! As Luke R. Bucci, Ph.D., Vice-President of research for Weider Nutrition Group, wrote in *Muscle & Fitness*: "Soy isn't just for vegetarians and people with milk allergies anymore."

I believe you'll agree I had ample reason to switch to Boca Burgers, but you may still have questions about bread. I thought the old-fashioned notion that bread is fattening had been put to rest. But as Anne Fletcher noted in *Eating Thin For Life*, the idea has been receiving renewed attention in the media, usually in connection with diet books such as *The Zone* or *Sugar Busters*. Countering the media hype, Fletcher reports that the eating habits of the masters of weight control she studied "are just the opposite." Says Fletcher: "Nearly half of the masters noted that they have bread at least two or three times a day."

"Bread... [is] good diet food provided that you eat it without butter," I wrote in *Ripped 2*. "I eat bread every day." That was true then, and it's true now.

Dr. Bob Arnot agrees with my advice on bread selection: "Your best, safest bet are the mixed grain and oat bran breads that are low in sugar and high in fiber." Even Barry Sears, author of The Zone, agrees on this point. He counsels, "If you do eat...bread, always use whole grain versions." Sears lists French bread and white bread as "rapid inducers of insulin." But he places whole-grain rye bread on his list of "reduced insulin secretion" foods with glycemic index scores between 30 and 50 percent.

> High-fiber breads are filling and satisfying without giving you too many calories. Bread—the right kind—is good diet food.

Again, high-fiber breads are filling and satisfying without giving you too many calories. Bread—the right kind—is good diet food. (See *Ripped 2* for an excellent study proving the value of bread for dieters.)

The BIG Stew

    3 cups frozen mixed vegetables
       (cauliflower, broccoli, zucchini, carrots)
    $1/2$ cup canned Santa Fe style beans
    3 ounces canned pink salmon or sardines (packed in water)
    2 cups water
    $1/2$ cup plain non-fat yogurt
    2 slices whole grain bread, toasted

This is my "new" favorite dinner. It's an upgrade of the vegetable stew with beef recipes in both *Ripped 3* and *Lean For Life*. The major changes are the addition of beans and the switch from extra-lean ground beef to fish. The calorie content is about the same, less than 600.

The choice of frozen vegetables mixtures available at supermarkets seems to get better every year. The California combo described here is one of my current favorites—Chinese stir-fry (broccoli, carrots, onions, green beans, sugar snap peas, celery, sweet red pepper and water chestnuts) is another—but any combination is fine. Check the ingredients to make sure no sugar or fatty sauce is added. I eat so many mixed vegetables that we buy the huge four-pound bag, which lasts me about a week.

Canned beans also come in many varieties. S&W Fine Foods (San Ramon, CA) is one of my favorite brands. Their "Simply Wonderful" slogan is right on target. The ingredients list on their beans is short and sweet, usually just prepared beans, water and a little sugar, salt and dehydrated onion. You'll find a much longer list of ingredients—including corn syrup, hydrogenated vegetable oil and monosodium glutamate—and more calories on some other brands. Most varieties of S&W brand beans contain 100 or less calories per one-half cup. The S&W Santa Fe style beans in this recipe have only 90 calories. Several of my other S&W brand favorites with their calorie content are as follows: black beans (70), white beans (80) and kidney beans (100).

Salmon and sardines are classified as "fatty fish." Believe it or not, that's a plus, as I'll explain shortly. Regular tuna fish (the full-fat variety), herring, lake trout and mackerel are also fatty fish, but canned salmon and sardines are easier to find. I use pink salmon, because it has about 20 percent fewer calories than red salmon, but still contains a meaningful amount of fat. I like sardines in mustard or tomato sauce, but I make sure it's packed in water, not oil. I also use canned tuna from time to time, but I've changed my mind on the fat content; I now look for the full-fat variety. Again, I make sure it's water-packed, not oil-packed.

Canned fish makes this recipe even easier to prepare than the beef stew in my earlier books. (I still eat beef occasionally because it's one of the best sources of iron.) Simply put the beans and fish into a big bowl—I use the same-sized bowl as breakfast—and stir them to-

> **The "fattest" fish has about the same amount of total fat as the leanest cuts of beef.**

gether. Add the vegetables and water. Stir again, and microwave for about six minutes. I use the time to toast the bread, take my vitamins, clean up and put everything away. Remove the stew from the microwave, stir in the nonfat yogurt and eat.

Comment

Don't be turned off by the term "fatty fish." As Artemis P. Simopoulos, M.D., explains in *The Omega Plan* (Harper Collins, 1998), "Unless you eat fatty fish two or more times a week you are likely to be deficient in [essential fatty acids]." Low-fat advocate Robert Pritikin says, "These fish contain a type of poly-unsaturated fat called Omega-3, which has been shown to reduce the tendency of blood to form clots." The Pritikin diet recommends $3^1/_2$ to 7 ounces of fatty fish per week. (The Pritikin "Best" choice diet allows one $3^1/_2$ ounce serving of lean beef, fowl or fish per day.)

Dr. Simopoulos says only fatty fish fill the bill, because "lean seafood, including cod, sole, flounder, crabs, and shrimp have about one-tenth the amount of Omega-3s as oily fish." What's more—get this—Simopoulos observes that the "fattest" fish has about the same amount of total fat as the leanest cuts of beef.

And don't forget the Japanese study discussed in the last chapter: Mice fed a 60% fish-oil diet were far leaner—in some cases "comparable to the difference in weight between a 225- and a 150-pound man," says Dr. Simopoulos—than mice fed a diet composed of lard or other types of fat.

> **The bottom line is that this dinner recipe is good for your waistline and good for the rest of you as well.**

As I said earlier, I'm enthusiastic about adding small portions of fatty fish to my diet on a regular basis. It's not likely to make me fat—and it might even make me leaner. Plus, a majority of studies have shown that consuming modest amounts of fatty fish protects against sudden death, according to *The Physician and Sportsmedicine* (May 1998).

The bottom line is that this dinner recipe is good for your waistline and good for the rest of you as well. The mixed vegetables are bulky and contain only 80 calories; the beans are low in calories, high in protein and slowly absorbed into your blood stream; and the salmon or sardines add taste and satiety, and may help you live longer and healthier.

The BIG stew is a good deal.

Smart Snacking

I've long been a smart snacker. All my books emphasize that snacking is a good thing for dieters. As I wrote in *Lean For Life*, "The truth is that snacking on the right kind of food keeps your appetite under control. It actually helps you stay lean." Frankly, I thought I knew just about all there was to know about snacking. But I learned some new facts about snacking in the course of researching this book—some that validate what I've been doing all along and others that have made me an even smarter snacker.

Everyone—from Jane Brody and Nancy Clark to Robert Pritikin, Barry Sears and Dr. Bob Arnot—recommends eating regular snacks. Prolific author and nutritionist Nancy Clark probably expressed the basic idea best. She said planned snacking is better than the "starve and stuff" routine. People who skip breakfast and eat next to nothing at lunch, usually stuff themselves in the evening. They eat practically non-stop from 5 o'clock until bedtime and end up gaining more weight than those who eat regular meals and snacks.

Dr. Bob Arnot's *Revolutionary Weight Control Program* includes an enlightening discussion of the work of Tufts University anthropology professor Stephen Bailey, Ph.D., on the history of snacking. "The whole notion of meals is an artificial and recent construction," says Dr. Bailey. Humans were made to eat continuously, according to Bailey.

Regular meals were spawned by the Industrial Revolution. Dr. Bailey says eating three times a day evolved to fit factory life. "If you look back in time, people grazed," says Bailey. "That's what our bodies are meant to do." He points out that our evolutionary cousins, the primates, don't have meals; chimps eat continuously. What's more, according to Bailey, young children who are not yet "socialized" tend to snack naturally, rather than eat three meals a day.

"If you snack you don't feel as hungry when you sit down to eat a 'meal'. As a result, you won't overeat."

Why is that important? Dr. Bailey explains: "If you snack you don't feel as hungry when you sit down to eat a 'meal'. As a result, you won't overeat. The norm today is that we fast between meals and suffer the consequences… We eat rapidly, and we eat a great deal." The underlying physiology is straightforward: "We don't have time for the food we eat to send hormonal signals to the brain that we have plenty of food in our stomach." We lose touch with the satiety response Dr. Chopra says we should rely on.

Eating three distinct and widely separated meals sets us up to gain weight, because the body perceives the time between meals as a famine. Dr. Bailey: "Your body slows down its metabolic rate and increases its efficiency at storing calories between meals, so that it can gorge during meals. Studies show you will gain more weight if you have the same number of calories and eat only one meal as opposed to distributing those same calories over four meals."

But there's also danger in snacking—because we've become conditioned to eating big meals. "People [must] remember that they've snacked and not go on to eat full meals as well," Dr. David Jenkins told Bob Arnot. That's where my put-everything-away rule comes to the rescue. Plan your meals and snacks—and put everything else away before you sit down to eat.

Okay, you say, snacks are good, but what should I eat?

First, don't buy into the conventional view that snacking means, well, snack food. Junk food and refined carbos, of course, are not the way to go. Clearly, candy, sweet rolls, soda pop and the like cause rebound hypoglycemia and practically insure that you will be ravenous at meal time.

There are basically two theories on the best snacks. One school emphasizes bulk and the other protein. Both discourage eating sugar and fat.

There are basically two theories on the best snacks. One school emphasizes bulk and the other protein. Both discourage eating sugar and fat.

Remember the index of food satisfaction developed by researchers at the University of Sidney? We discussed it in the last chapter. Dr. Susanne Holt and her colleagues measured the capacity of different foods to provide fullness, or satiety. As you'll recall, they found that foods high in sugar and fat rate low on the "satiety index" and that foods high in fiber and water and protein-rich foods provide the highest levels of satisfaction.

Consistent with this finding, James Stubbs, Ph.D., of the Rowett Research Institute in Aberdeen Scotland, proposes that there is a hierarchy of satiating effects of foods based on the storage capacity of the body. Stubbs says there is almost no storage capacity for protein, a limited storage capacity for carbohydrates and an almost unlimited capacity to store fat. He says, quite logically, that the body burns fuels it can't store first and is satiated in the same order. "[Stubbs' work] shows that protein is more satiating than carbohydrates, which is more satiating than fat," says Dr. Bob Arnot.

Dr. Stubbs suggests snacking on protein to quell the appetite, because there's something in protein that quickly signals the brain that you've had enough. Fat, on the other hand, doesn't work, because there's nothing in fat to kill your appetite. As Robert Pritikin explains in *Weight Loss Breakthrough*, "Our ancestors had to get as much fat into their systems as they could because there was no telling when they would have another feast....Gorging on fat—with it's abundance of calories—became a key to survival."

Dr. Arnot cautions that small amounts of protein don't work. One hundred calories or more, however, act as a powerful appetite suppressant. "In one study," Arnot relates, "obese subjects decreased the number of calories they ate at the next meal by

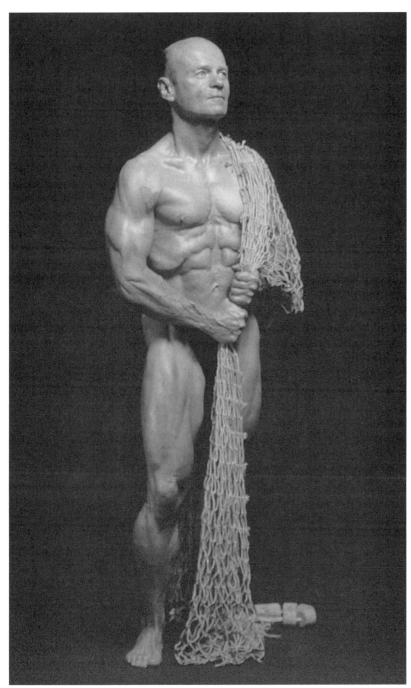

Carol suggested this net pose during our latest photo shoot. It shows my 60-year-old physique to good advantage. Eating regular, planned snacks helped me achieve this condition. *Photo by Pat Berrett*.

19 percent when they ate 155 calories of protein compared to the same amount of carbohydrates."

I've found that preloading on protein is a great way to curb the appetite and stay in control of how much I eat. First thing in the morning, I have a glass of skimmed milk with one half teaspoon (2.5g) of creatine monohydrate added. This allows me to start the day feeling good and under control. Milk, with its ample supply of protein, keeps me satisfied while I read the morning newspaper and fix my breakfast. In addition, I frequently have a glass of skimmed milk as a preemptive strike before I go out to eat or to a social gathering. That makes it easy to keep my hands off the bread and butter while I'm waiting to be served in a restaurant, and helps insure that I select wisely from the tempting tidbits served at social gatherings. Beans also work well for this purpose. One half cup of black beans and a little milk makes an amazingly satisfying mid-afternoon snack. When I'm trying to get another hour of productive work out of myself at the end of a long day, I often stir a heaping tablespoonful of protein powder into a glass of skimmed milk; that picks me up nicely until dinner. (To compensate, I skip the yogurt and cut back on the beans in my Big stew.)

I also subscribe to the bulk theory of snacking. *The Pritikin Weight Loss Breakthrough* says, "Fiber and water provide bulk, which fills you up.... Fiber and water have no calories, which means that you experience fullness, without gaining weight." The foods that provide the most bulk, with the least fat and sugar are generally vegetables, fruit and whole grains.

Robert Pritikin himself eats frequent, bulky snacks. For example, after a breakfast of oatmeal with fruit and a half hour to 40 minutes on the treadmill, he has a fruit snack on the way to work. After he's been at work for an hour of so, he usually has a cup of vegetable soup at his desk. "The soup," says Pritikin, "gives me real satisfaction on very few calories [and] provides me with lots of energy so I'm well fortified for the morning." Pritikin's list of "Best" snacks includes raw veggies, baked sweet potatoes, fresh fruit and bean dip.

My favorite fruit snack is an apple, which I eat seeds and all, everything but the stem. I frequently have an apple at mid-morning, after my walk. I always have a mid-afternoon snack, usually one of Carol's homemade scones (see recipe below) or some beans and a slice of whole grain bread. What's more, I never skip my bedtime snack, which is usually some version of the fruit and yogurt mixture I have for lunch and another one of Carol's scones.

I never starve and stuff, to use Nancy Clark's phrase. Like

our ancient ancestors, I eat throughout the day. Take my cue. Eat regular, planned snacks.

(You'll find more snack suggestions in *Ripped 3* and *Lean For Life*.)

Carol's Scone Recipe

The following is the scone recipe I have been baking at our house for about four years. It is a variation of a recipe from the book *Secrets of Fat Free Baking* by Sandra Woodruff, R.D. (Avery Publishing Group, 1994).

It took a lot of experimentation to find a recipe that suited our needs for a planned snack. We wanted to feel free to have a good-tasting treat without worrying about huge numbers of calories, and it needed to be satisfying. Satisfaction after eating is important. If you don't feel satisfied then you just want to eat more. This scone requires some time to chew, and it's that chewing which is part of the eating satisfaction. And, since it contains honey, a concentrated sweet, it needed to have protein in it to slow absorption and keep the blood sugar balanced. My version has an extra cup of oats, 1 tablespoon more egg substitute, and 1 tablespoon more buttermilk than the original recipe, because we like a larger, less sweet scone. Feel free to change it around to suit your needs.

Clarence usually has one of these scones in mid-afternoon with milk or yogurt. I like mine late in the day with hot, non-fat soy milk to which I add almond extract or ground cardamom for extra flavor.

Cinnamon Oat Scones

$1^1/_2$ cup whole wheat pastry flour or unbleached flour
2 cups rolled oats
1 tablespoon baking powder
$^1/_4$ cup honey, brown rice syrup or barley malt
$^1/_3$ cup raisins
4 tablespoons (or more) Egg Beaters or other egg substitute
$^1/_4$ cup plus 3 tablespoons (or more) nonfat buttermilk (or in a
    pinch, yogurt)
$^1/_2$ tsp. ground cinnamon
$^1/_2$ to 1 tsp. almond extract (optional)

In one bowl, combine flour, oats, baking powder, raisins,
    and cinnamon.
In another bowl, combine honey, egg substitute, buttermilk
    and almond flavoring.
Mix the dry and wet ingredients together and form into a round

flat circle with your hands (about 7 inches across). The dough should be fairly stiff but should hold together. Add more liquid or oats depending on your needs.

I bake this on a baking sheet lined with parchment paper. This way there is virtually no clean up. Parchment paper can be purchased at any gourmet store or any large health food store. If you don't have it, simply coat a baking sheet with a cooking spray.

Cut the circle into 12 pieces, coat with skim milk to brown the scones, and bake at 375° for 20–23 minutes until slightly brown.

Store in the refrigerator.

"It's best to leave a little bit in the gym so you can go back the next day and pick it up and start all over again."
—*Bill Pearl*, bodybuilding legend

CHAPTER FOUR

The Ripped Training Philosophy Revisited

An Important Chapter

This is an important chapter. As you know by now, this is more than a "how to" book. We cover the "how," but we also deal extensively with the "why." This chapter is about the "why" of training. It will put you on a sound footing, both psychologically and physiologically. What's more, it will provide you with the knowledge you need to keep progressing, literally forever.

> **This is an important chapter. Stick with me. I promise you won't be sorry.**

Obviously, that's a tall order. As a glance at the table of contents will indicate, we cover a lot of ground in this chapter. Master the information presented here, however, and you'll have an elite understanding of the significant issues in training. Stick with me. I promise you won't be sorry.

The Exercise Challenge

Diet and exercise have one thing in common. Long-term success in both depends on short-term satisfaction. Enjoyment, believe it or not, is the key ingredient in any really successful exercise plan. That doesn't mean the program must be easy. To the contrary, productive exercise is often brutally hard. What it does mean is that the regimen must be satisfying. Training satisfaction, of course, comes from progress. It's a virtuous circle. Progress is satisfying, and training satisfaction motivates you to keep striving—and progressing. What it boils down to is that progress leads to more progress. Nothing succeeds like success.

Sounds like a riddle, I know, but it's really not. It simply means the exercise challenge is to make every workout a productive and positive experience. Success comes when you enjoy the process.

Focus on the Present

Expecting too much too soon stymies many bodybuilding programs. I frequently hear from people—usually beginners—who expect immediate results. One fellow who had been training for "about one month" wanted me to tell him how to "develop big arms and chest fast." Another wanted "dramatic gains in lean muscle mass." He wrote, "I am interested in building a physique like [many times Mr. Universe] Bill Pearl." These fellows, of course, are getting way ahead of themselves. If they don't lower their sights, at least initially, they will soon be ex-bodybuilders.

A much better approach for these young men—and for most people—is to focus on the here and now. Keep in mind that today was yesterday's tomorrow. As the famous doctor-runner-philosopher George Sheehan wrote in *Personal Best*, "Here in this very day is our happiness." If you make it a point to enjoy today's workout, you'll be motivated to train again tomorrow. Workout by workout, step by step, you'll keep moving down the road of progress.

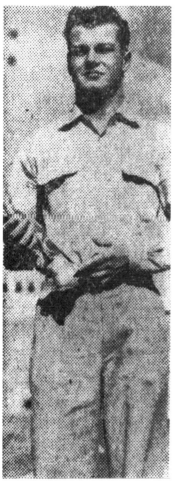

I started training with weights when I was about 13—and never stopped. I had an excellent beginning, because I found a sport I enjoyed.

Find Your Sport

In *Running To Win*, George Sheehan acknowledged that some people find running a bore. Not everyone is cut out for the marathon. I'm certainly not. The same holds true for weight training. Sheehan, however, believed strongly that this should not be an excuse for sedentary living. "We are meant to be athletes, not spectators," he said. "And we must find our sport."

It won't take long to decide whether you like lifting. I knew right away. Like most people, my body responded readily to weight

Fortunately, my training brought success early on. I knew right away that lifting was my forte. Strength training gave me the power to win the state high school pentathlon championship. This fuzzy newspaper photo shows me on the victory platform.

training. By the time I was a sophomore in high school I could lift more than my friends. The next year, weight training gave me the power to win the state high school pentathlon championship. And when I was a senior, I won my first city Olympic weight lifting championship. So I knew weights were my thing.

That doesn't mean, of course, that you have to be a champion to enjoy lifting. Just give yourself a little time; you'll know. If pumping iron starts to feel good and you like the changes you see in the mirror, weight training is probably for you. If not, try something else. Find your sport.

Develop the Self

As I urged in chapter one, compete with yourself. Philosophers over the ages have generally agreed on the basic rule for a happy life: Develop the self. As George Sheehan put it in *Personal Best*, "To be happy, grow." He added this important corollary: "We each have a role to play—our own." Our happiness—and ultimately our success—depends on the extent to which we play that role to the best of our ability.

> **It may surprise you to learn that more bodybuilders fail because of overtraining than undertraining. If you are not making progress and dread your next workout, you're probably training too much.**

As the young man who wrote to me needs to understand, few of us have the genetics of a Bill Pearl. Nevertheless, we can all improve. Most beginners can, in fact, improve dramatically—but not overnight. It takes time. You must persist.

Make slow, steady improvement the focus of your training. Don't compare yourself to anyone else. Judge progress based on your previous condition. Make each training session a positive experience, and your long-term success will be assured. Remember, your most important competitor, the only one that really counts, is you.

The Path to Progress

Don't overtrain or undertrain. Both extremes cause lack of progress, which is usually the reason why people throw in the towel. You need positive feedback to stay motivated. Results are what make training worthwhile. The path to progress is narrow, with overtraining on one side and undertraining on the other. Get off the path and you may be sidetracked for ever.

It may surprise you to learn that more bodybuilders fail because of overtraining than undertraining. If you are not making progress and dread your next workout, you're probably training too much. That's why we'll talk a lot about the importance of rest in this book. In bodybuilding less training often brings better results; less is often more.

No "Best Way"

As I wrote in *Lean For Life*, "There is no single 'best way' to train." After a time the body stops responding to any program. To keep making improvements—especially if you are an advanced trainer—you have to continually change your routine. A new routine sets off a new adaptation response in the body and, presto, gains begin again.

What's more, training the same way all the time is no fun. "Boredom kills more fitness programs than any other villain," Terry and Jan Todd observed in their classic *Lift Your Way To Youthful Fitness*. "The best medicine for dull, monotonous training is variety," says Dr. Tudor O. Bompa, revolutionary strength training authority and author of *Serious Strength Training* (Human Kinetics, 1998). "Remember, both your mind and your body become bored," counsels Bompa.

Variation is a basic theme of this book. We'll be discussing a form of training called periodization. The advantage of this system is that no two workouts are ever the same. Training is done in constantly changing phases and cycles. Every workout you either vary the exercises, the poundages, or the number of repetitions. The basic idea is that you push until you almost, but not quite, reach a plateau or sticking point, and then you back off and begin again, with a different training emphasis. Importantly, you are always moving forward and almost never fail. That makes training enjoyable.

Enjoyment, as we said, is ultimately the key to progress. Remember, enjoy the process.

Now, let's turn to the main driver of every successful training program: overload.

The Basic Principle

"In weight training, there's only one scientific fact: progressive overloads build muscle." That quote from New York Giants strength and conditioning coach John Dunn appeared in the August 17, 1998 *Sports Illustrated*, and it's right on target. There are many theories in the ever-evolving field of weight training, but overload is the one principle that's beyond dispute. It simply says to increase strength and lean body mass you must continually challenge yourself to lift more than you have before. Do that, gradually and progressively, and you will become bigger and stronger.

The concept is simple, but the execution, especially when you move beyond the beginners stage, is often problematic. It's difficult, of course, to force yourself to go into the gym, workout after workout, and lift progressively heavier weights. But the problem is more involved than that. As in the case of dieting, willpower alone is not the answer.

The task of continually overloading the muscles is more complex than it might appear. It's not as straightforward as suggested by the story from Greek mythology of Milo of Croton who became the strongest man in the world by lifting and carrying a calf every day until it grew into a full-grown bull.

As indicated in the last section, unrelenting pressure to increase training load and intensity eventually overcomes the ability of the body and mind to adapt. One must periodically back off in response to what Tudor O. Bompa, Ph.D., currently a professor at York University in Toronto, Ontario, Canada, calls the physiological and psychological "crisis of fatigue." Says Bompa, whose groundbreaking theory of periodization, introduced in 1963, helped his native Romania and the Eastern Bloc countries dominate international sports in the 1970s and 1980s: "A period of unloading... serves as a reprieve for the body, so it can adapt to the new, more intense stressors and regenerate itself in preparation for yet another load increase."

> **Boiled down to its essence, periodization is simply organized variation of the training program.**

Periodization

I believe my book *Ripped 3*, published in 1986, was the first to apply periodization to bodybuilding. Boiled down to its essence, periodization is simply organized variation of the training program. We've all noticed how something as simple as changing an exercise or a hand or foot position can freshen a routine; it makes you sore and kicks the body into another round of adaptation. You've probably also had the experience of missing a workout or two or perhaps being forced to lighten up for a time because of a minor injury. What happened when you resumed normal training? You expect to find yourself deconditioned and weaker—after all, conventional wisdom says that detraining starts within 96 hours—but more often than not—you're actually stronger!

Periodization puts lessons learned from such experiences to work in an organized way. Instead of trying to blast through the sticking points we all encounter, as I put it in *Ripped 3*, "You push for a while, back off, and then push again, each time peaking a little higher than before." You start a new training phase with a new repetition range and different poundages, or perhaps a change of exercises or manner of performance—and your progress takes off again.

As we'll see in the training routines, there are many variations of periodization. The one constant, however, in all periodization plans is change.

Remember that your goal is to get in shape and stay there year after year. Understanding how to alter the pattern of your training through periodization will enable you to continue training successfully over long periods of time. As an athlete who has trained continually for over 45 years, I recommend you give it a try.

By the way, overload and periodization apply to aerobic conditioning as well as weight training.

In the rest of this chapter, we are going to discuss some of the most hotly debated aspects of weight training. They have to do with how much you should train and how much you should rest (the overload and adaptation cycle).

(See *Ripped 2* for a more technical discussion of overload and the role of intensity in triggering adaptation.)

Stress and Rest

As mentioned earlier, many—perhaps most—bodybuilders overtrain; they train too much or too often. Bodybuilders become so fixated on intensity or getting a pump that they forget the other side of the growth equation: rest and recovery.

As I explained in *Ripped 2*, rest is very important to the success of any training program. Muscle growth is stimulated by hard training (overload), but you must permit growth to occur by resting. George Sheehan, the fitness philosopher, may have put it best: "The body can be trained to greater performance by induced stress. But the amount of stress and the time allowed for recovery are critical to the success of the process."

> **Expert opinion on optimum training frequency varies widely. Train too often, some emphasize, and you will short-circuit supercompensation, but others, equally adamant, warn that if you wait too long, the opportunity for growth will be lost.**

The ability of the body to recover from exercise is limited. Hard training will get you nowhere unless you follow up with enough rest to permit growth to take place. Without adequate rest, your body is forced to use all of its recovery ability just to restore itself. For growth to take place,

65

the body must be given time to not only recover the energy expended in training but for growth as well. This is called supercompensation; the body not only returns to its preworkout state, but also prepares itself to better withstand the stress of the next workout by becoming bigger and stronger.

Unfortunately, the process of recovery and supercompensation is not fully understood, which gives rise to the hot debate. How much should you train? How much rest should you have between training sessions? Not surprisingly, as I detail below, expert opinion on optimum training frequency varies widely. Train too often, some emphasize, and you will short-circuit supercompensation, but others, equally adamant, warn that if you wait too long, the opportunity for growth will be lost.

The experts generally can be grouped into two camps: those favoring long, fast-paced sessions spaced a day or two apart (volume training) and those who prefer short, very hard sessions spaced much further apart (high intensity training).

In *Serious Strength Training*, Dr. Bompa writes: "[Recreational] bodybuilders will probably get the best results from training three times a week with a total body routine. Less training frequency than this would decrease efficiency and reduce the necessary adaptive response." According to Bompa, serious strength athletes and competitive bodybuilders should train 4-6 times a week using a split routine, training each body part every second day or so. He seriously questions whether training each muscle group twice each week—or "even worse," once—is adequate. "In our opinion, neither is enough," he states emphatically.

(Even more extreme, Bulgarian Olympic Weightlifters, who along with the Russians, dominated competitive lifting for many years, trained heavy four or five times *a day*, but erogenic aids— steroids, for example—may have been used to enhance their recovery capacity.)

At the other end of the spectrum, high-intensity-training advocate Mike Mentzer, the 1978 Mr. Universe and a former professional bodybuilder, maintains that recovery capacity is genetically mediated and that some people will do best by training only once every two or three weeks! In *Heavy Duty 2*, Mentzer suggests that people begin by training once every 4 or 5 days, using a split routine consisting of only 3 to 5 very hard work sets in each workout. "After 6-9 months, depending on genetics and previous training history," Mentzer says, "you will be training only once every 6-7 days, or even less frequently."

Why is there so much disagreement? Even more perplexing, why do both schools of training produce outstanding results?

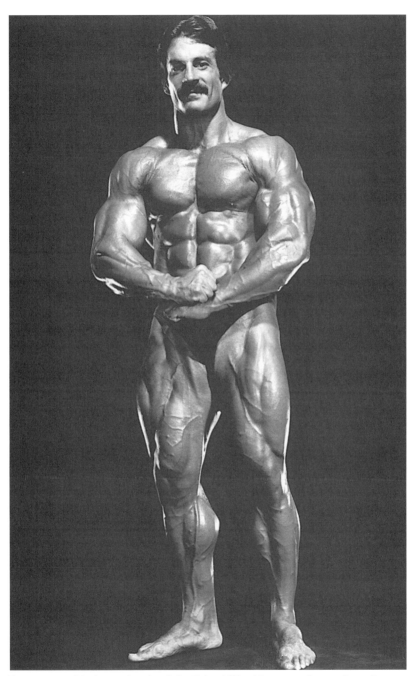

Former world champion bodybuilder Mike Mentzer, shown here in top shape, is probably the leading proponent of infrequent, high intensity training. He suggests that people begin training once every 4 or 5 days. *Photo courtesy of Mike Mentzer.*

The answer, I believe, lies in two different theories of supercompensation: wound healing and energy depletion. What's more, I believe that both theories are probably correct. Both camps will probably consider that an outlandish statement, so I'll explain. I'll also tell you which side I favor, and why.

Understanding both theories will allow you to choose the type of training best for your goals and your temperament and will clear up a lot of confusion about how to train.

HIT and Volume, Two Different Models of Supercompensation

Six-time Mr. Olympia Dorian Yates belongs to the high-intensity school of training (HIT), which is compatible with the wound healing or muscle cell damage theory. Led by Mike Mentzer, the first and only bodybuilder ever to receive a perfect score in the amateur world championship, the HIT people believe in very hard, very brief and infrequent training. Mentzer directed my attention to the wound healing theory of supercompensation.

The high-volume school, on the other hand, is probably favored by the majority of North American bodybuilders, including the highly respected Bill Pearl. They believe in high-set, frequent training. They go for the pump. Dr. Bompa, who I put in the volume camp, strongly backs the energy depletion model of supercompensation, at least for muscle hypertrophy (enlargement).

Let's start with energy depletion and how it explains the effectiveness of high-volume training. Energy depletion is simply that state, as detailed below, when the muscle has used up its energy stores and you cannot exercise any more. (We'll discuss the wound healing theory in the next section.)

"The key element in hypertrophy training," says Bompa, "is the cumulative effect of the total number of sets."

"Supercompensation can only be achieved... if work and regeneration are timed perfectly," says Bompa. Here's why.

Fast, pump-type training, with 60 seconds or less rest between sets, depletes the muscle's energy stores (ATP/CP and glycogen), causing fatigue and temporarily reduces your ability to train. The short rest periods prevent energy stores from being completely replaced between sets. After a few sets, energy depletion, along with lactic acid accumulation, effectively shut the muscle down.

"The key element in hypertrophy training," says Bompa, "is the cumulative effect of the total number of sets." The cumulative exhaustion of the energy stores in the muscles threatens

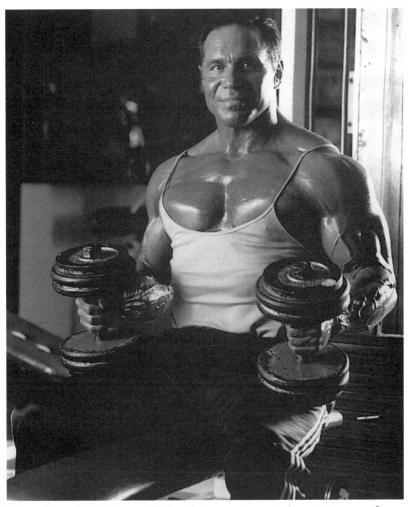

Many times Mr. Universe Bill Pearl, shown here at about 58 years of age, trains two hours a day, six days a week, using a split routine. Bill changes his workouts regularly. *Photo by Chris Lund, courtesy of Bill Pearl.*

the body's survival, and it is forced to adapt after training. The body responds by replenishing the lost energy stores, first to normal levels, and then by creating additional reserves. "This energy rebound puts the athlete into a state of supercompensation and gives him or her the energy needed to train even harder," Bompa explains. "This is essential for adaptation to training, and consequently, for improved muscle size." Muscle growth "occurs as a result of increasing the [energy reserves] in the muscle cells and activating protein metabolism." So the body has rested, the muscle's energy has been restored and, in fact, increased (supercompensated). In addition, the size of the muscle has increased because of the extra shorted energy.

If you train too often, Bompa warns, the energy stores are depleted again before supercompensation and growth can occur. On the other hand, says Bompa, "If the time between two workouts is too long, the supercompensation will fade away, resulting in little, if any, improvement." That's why he believes training frequency is so critical. According to Bompa, the optimal recovery period for this type of training is, you guessed it, about 48 hours.

"When the body is rested and full of fuel, it can be pushed to heights never dreamed of before," Bompa maintains, enthusiastically. "By training this way, one can expect supercompensation [muscle growth] to occur every 2–4 days."

Wow, sounds great. But even the proponents of volume training say there's a downside. Bompa says most North American bodybuilders use only the energy depletion system to increase muscle size—and they succeed. But the muscle developed using this type of hypertrophy training "is usually not chronic [lasting], because the growth is largely due to fluid displacement within the muscles rather than a thickening of muscle fibers." As explained in *Ripped 3*, the muscle fibers that thicken are primarily the fast-twitch fibers.

This deficiency can be corrected using what Bompa calls the "maximum load method," which has many parallels to HIT. It utilizes high intensity and long rest intervals to stimulate the maximum number of fast-twitch muscle fibers.

The main points of disagreement between the two schools of training (volume and HIT) are the optimum number of sets and the frequency of training.

There is broad agreement that high-intensity training builds good quality muscle. As just indicated, Dr. Bompa believes high-intensity training—sets of 3 to 8 reps using maximum poundages and rest intervals of 3-5 minutes—is necessary for complete development.

Charles Poliquin, another well known proponent of volume training, also recommends including maximum poundages and long rest intervals in the overall training regimen. In *The Poliquin Principles* (Dayton Writers Group, 1997), he says this type of training is "great for creating hypertrophy by favoring growth of the contractile proteins."

The main points of disagreement between the two schools of training (volume and HIT) are the optimum number of sets and the frequency of training. As we've seen, Dr. Bompa favors training each muscle group about three times each week. He recommends 4 to 12 sets per muscle group.

Poliquin is more moderate, and closer to the high-intensity camp (Mentzer) on training frequency. He says, "For most individuals, three to four days' rest between workouts for the same bodypart appears to be good advice." Poliquin, however, advocates more reps and sets than Mentzer. For hypertrophy, he generally recommends 6-20 reps and 3-6 sets per exercise. While definitely not a Mentzer fan, Poliquin believes that both high volume and high-intensity build muscle, but for different reasons. Like me, Poliquin says, "Both camps are right!"

Now, let's look at the wound healing theory of recovery and how it supports HIT and infrequent workouts.

The Wound Healing Model

I've long been a supporter—and practitioner—of short, hard and infrequent weight training. But until Mike Mentzer called an article by David Staplin to my attention recently, I'd never considered wound healing as a model for muscle recovery and adaptation. It is easy to grasp the wound wound healing idea if you simply think of it the way you do if you cut yourself. The wound healing model relates to the time it takes the cut to heal. Staplin applies that concept to muscles subjected to training.

Dave Staplin has taught cell biology, anatomy and physiology at the University of Minnesota and St. Paul Technical College and is a lifetime bodybuilder. His article, "Understanding Recovery: A Wound Healing Model," on Mike's web site (mikementzer.com), has given me a new perspective on supercompensation. Staplin appears to be one of the few people (perhaps the only one) doing serious research on this very new topic. His work suggests, to me at least, that there may be a substantial difference in the time course of recovery and supercompensation for the two principal types of bodybuilding training. Could it be that Bompa and Mentzer are both substantially correct about optimum training frequency—for their chosen brand of training?

Staplin believes the wound healing process, especially the inflammatory response, provides a good model for studying and understanding muscle recovery. He explains that high-intensity training damages the muscle cells and, importantly, that the degree of damage depends on the intensity of the exercise. "The higher the intensity, the greater the damage," says Staplin. "It is the process of healing this damage which then makes the muscle cell larger and stronger."

Healing requires a number of steps. Significantly, each step must occur in a specific sequence and, of course, each step takes time. One of the steps, inflammation, actually causes further damage.

While the exact healing mechanism is unclear and still being studied, there appears to be six steps, some of which are quite technical and meaningful only to an exercise physiologist. The key points in the process, however, are pretty straightforward.

Muscle cell damage, the first step, causes an inflammatory response (steps 2–4), which in turn causes further damage (step 5). The damage caused by the inflammatory response may continue for several days. Delayed-onset muscle soreness, which can last up to 7 days or even longer, is thought to be one effect of the acute inflammatory process.

Very significantly, it is only after steps 1–5 have been completed that step 6, tissue regeneration (rebuilding of the muscle), can begin.

Like the process of energy replacement after volume training, the muscle cell must first rebuild to preworkout levels. "Only then, and only IF allowed further time, will [the muscle cell] supercompensate and build up to levels greater than before," Staplin emphasizes.

How long does the entire process take? It depends on the degree of trauma, or in our case, the intensity of the exercise and other related and individual factors, according to Staplin. But the entire 6-step process can take—get this—"from 5 days to over 6 weeks."

"This has profound implications regarding frequency of training!" Staplin says. "The more intense your training, the longer you must allow for recovery."

Profound implications, indeed.

As mentioned, Staplin is a serious bodybuilder. Not only has he thought and read about the subject, he's experimented with different training frequencies in his own workouts. He sustained a severe injury several years ago, which forced him to take an extended layoff from training. As a result, his weight dropped from 205 to 180. Dave tells me that in the course of rehabilitating himself, over a period of more than a year, his training slowly evolved from three times a week (two upper body and one lower, 5–6 worksets per workout), to twice a week and eventually to once every 7–10 days. "I managed to get up to about 210 pounds," Dave says. After that, however, he admits that he got a little carried away and overshot the mark. "As an experiment, I tried four negative-only workouts spaced three weeks apart.... My bodyweight went from about 210 to 227. Unfortunately, the majority of this gain was an increase in body fat."

Looking back now, on his personal experience and his research, Dave says, "I think the wound healing model is an interesting and valid idea when looking at the response of muscle cells to intense training." Like any good scientist, however, he cautions that there is still much to learn. For example, Staplin says, "There is more to training stimulus and recovery than just responses at the cellular level."

Be that as it may, based on Staplin's admittedly embryonic work, it seems logical to assume—or at least speculate—that it takes longer, perhaps considerably longer, to repair the damage caused to muscle cells by high-intensity training than it does to replenish the energy stores depleted by fast, volume training. I believe it is possible, perhaps likely, that a bodybuilder can recover and supercompensate from volume training in 2 to 4 days, as Bompa and Poliquin suggest, but that the process takes up to 3 weeks in the case of HIT training. How else do we explain the magnificent physiques developed by both systems of training?

So, where does that leave us? On a personal level, I've never done fast, volume training; it never appealed to me. But I've done plenty of very intense aerobic work, which is similar to volume bodybuilding. (We'll discuss high-intensity aerobics later in this chapter.) I feel exhausted after hard aerobics, but not inflamed like I do for days after high-intensity weight workouts. I can recover from a very hard aerobics session in a day or two but, as the wound healing model would predict, it takes me a full week and sometimes more to fully recover from high-intensity weight sessions.

As already stipulated, we still have a lot to learn about the exact process of supercompensation following exercise. Nevertheless, it makes sense that lactic acid accumulation, which is part and parcel of fast volume training (and high-intensity aerobics), protects the muscle cells from damage and, therefore, shortens the time required for recovery. Remember, you can train hard or you can train long, but you can't do both. The two types of training are mutually exclusive.

Remember too that Dr. Bompa and Charles Poliquin, both volume training advocates, agree that high-intensity training—and not volume training—promotes growth of the muscle fibers. The body has many protective mechanisms. Perhaps volume training, specifically the fatigue products it generates, functions to protect the muscle cells from damage.

> **In short, HIT may inflict greater damage on the muscle cells by shortcircuiting the body's protective mechanisms—and may therefore require a substantially longer recovery period. On the other hand, the recovery time for volume training, because it stresses the energy stores—and protects the contractile fibers—may be much shorter.**

Brief, very hard training, on the other hand, is by its very nature calculated to inflict maximum possible damage on the contractile fibers. Dr. Bompa, in effect, makes that point when he says, "One of the main objectives of [high-intensity] training is to teach the body to eliminate CNS [central nervous system] inhibition."

In short, HIT may inflict greater damage on the muscle cells by shortcircuiting the body's protective mechanisms—and may therefore require a substantially longer recovery period. On the other hand, the recovery time for volume training, because it stresses the energy stores—and protects the contractile fibers—may be much shorter.

Based on current knowledge, personal experience and common sense, my best guess is that both camps are essentially correct on optimum frequency—for their respective schools of training.

Think about it.

I'm a HIT Man

I've already said that I'm in the high intensity camp. I tried high-set training when I first turned to bodybuilding in my late 30s, but it didn't take long to decide it wasn't for me. I wrote in *Ripped*: One of the lessons I learned in 1979 was that "short, intense training" produces the "best results."

In 1979, I reduced total sets per workout by one half—cutting back to an average of four sets per body part—and began training my body only once every four days. I wrote in *Ripped* that these changes "resulted in more intense workouts... With more rest, fewer sets, and shorter workouts, I could make every set count. I was no longer, consciously or unconsciously, forced to hold back on early sets so I would be able to finish my workout."

Even then I sensed that multiple sets challenge energy reserves more than the contractile power of the muscle itself. I wrote: "Once the muscle is warmed up and ready for maximum effort, there's no point [in doing] a number of intermediate sets, [which] don't challenge the muscle and stimulate growth, but they do reduce the energy that can be put into the heaviest set, the set which does stimulate growth."

Then as now, doing only one or two work sets was getting off the beaten path. I said, "It's important to note I don't agree with the usual practice. I skip the non-productive sets. I go right to the set that really counts."

Continuing the discussion in *Ripped 2*, I wrote: "I don't rush my workouts at the expense of training intensity. I take enough

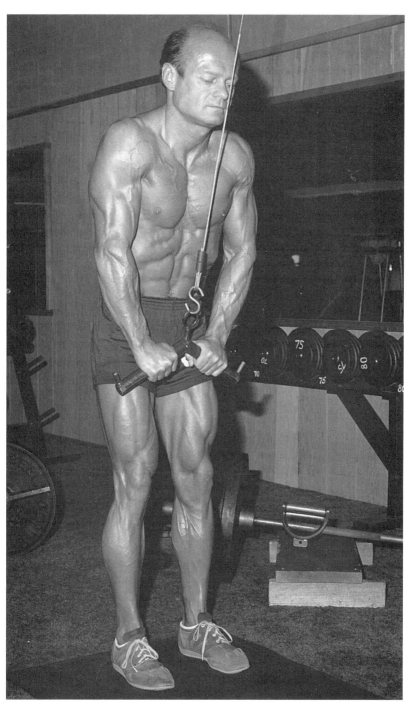

One reason I'm still training—and gaining—after all these years is that I've always tried to train as efficiently as possible. *Photo by Bill Reynolds.*

rest so that I can put maximum effort into [every set]." Clearly, I knew that rushing from set to set, as Bompa suggests, makes it impossible to challenge the maximum number of muscle fibers. You can train long or hard, but you can't do both.

So I had it more than half right. I was correct that low-volume, high-intensity training is the best way to promote growth of the contractile fibers. (I was still training too often, however.) I knew that high sets challenged my energy reserves; but I didn't realize that properly timed volume training, with short rest periods between sets, actually builds a different kind of muscle. I didn't know that fast-paced, high-set training promotes hypertrophy through increased energy substrate storage. It didn't dawn on me that some combination of HIT and volume training might be the way to build maximum muscle mass.

Still, had I known then what I know now, I'm not sure I would have trained differently. Here's why.

I hinted at the reason in *Ripped*. I said that high-intensity, infrequent training not only challenged my muscle fibers to the max, "it also [made] my training sessions more satisfying and more interesting."

I like to train. I must, I've been at it for over 45 years. But I've never wanted to spend my life in the gym. I definitely don't want to be *required* to train six days a week. A system of training that says my gains will fade if I don't pump every body part every few days is not my idea of fun. That reminds me of the old English treadmills that were formerly used to discipline prison inmates. I'm glad I didn't take that path. It would very likely have run me out of the gym years ago.

Al Vermeil, the highly regarded strength and conditioning coach for the Chicago Bulls, emphasized that high-volume, low-intensity training builds mass, but does not do a very good job of increasing force production.

One reason I'm still training—and gaining—after all these years is that I've always tried to train as efficiently as possible. I don't enjoy doing the same exercise over and over; I find it boring. I'd much prefer to warm up, really drill a set, and move on to the next exercise. I like to get the job done in the gym, and then get on with my life. Brief, intense and infrequent training fills the bill.

Another reason for my preference is physiological. Brief, high-intensity training builds functional muscle, and volume bodybuilding tends not to. Al Vermeil, the highly regarded strength and conditioning coach for the Chicago Bulls, emphasized this point recently in an unpublished research paper. Vermeil stressed that high-volume, low-intensity training builds mass,

76

but does not do a very good job of increasing force production. As explained earlier, traditional high-set bodybuilding increases the noncontractile fibers; the muscle size produced is mainly due to fluid buildup. The problem, says Vermeil, is that "relative strength doesn't improve so the increased mass has a negative effect on the speed of movement and jumping ability." By contrast, high-intensity, low-volume training increases the size and strength of the fast twitch muscle fibers. The result, says Vermeil, is "functional hypertrophy." In other words, HIT training builds muscle you can use.

Yes, I'm a HIT man, as indicated by my personal routine in the next chapter. But you'll also see there a routine which combines volume and high intensity to get the best of both worlds.

Now, lets turn to a discussion of whole body strength training (athletic-type training), which may be new to many of you. This includes Snatches, Cleans and Squats.

Athletic-Type Strength Training

I learned early on that weight training makes one a better athlete. In *The Lean Advantage 3*, I told how in 1954 a "secret weapon" helped me to out-jump everyone in a state high school fitness competition. I began my athletic career by winning the New Mexico State High School Pentathlon Championship, a five-event contest consisting of push-ups, chin-ups, jump reach, bar vault and 300-yd shuttle run. Weight training gave me a leg up on the competition. As I recall, I won every event but the shuttle run, but I had a special advantage in the jump reach, a test of leg and hip power. I was doing a type of exercise untried by the other guys. My secret weapon was what Dr. Pat O'Shea, author of *Quantum Strength & Power Training* (Patrick Books, 1996), now calls "athletic-type strength training."

Even though I was only a junior in high school, I had already been doing Snatches, Clean & Jerks, High Pulls and Squats for a number of years. I used heavy weights and low reps (1–5) in these full-range, multiple-joint lifting movements. These lifts gave me the explosive power in the thighs, hips and lower back to jump higher than the others. Today, because they stress the leaping muscles of the body, exercises like these form the core of the training program of many, perhaps most, athletes—in all sports. The NFL, the NBA, college programs, and even high school athletes use these full body movements. That wasn't always the case, however. In keeping with the prevailing wisdom of the time, my high school coach discouraging me from doing any type of weight training. I had to lift on my own, at home.

The turning point in the general acceptance of lifting came a couple of years later with the publication of a book by Jim Murray and Peter V. Karpovich, M.D. The book was *Weight Training in Athletics*, published by Prentice Hall in 1956. Jim Murray was a former managing editor of *Strength & Health* magazine and Dr. Karpovich was a professor at Springfield College in Massachusetts and one of the most respected exercise physiologists of his time. As Murray recounted recently in *Iron Game History*, Karpovich, a non-lifter, once believed—along with most physicians, coaches and physical educators—that weight training made a person slow, inflexible and clumsy, in a word "musclebound."

I read this landmark book soon after it came out—it's still in my library—and remember getting a kick out of Dr. Karpovich's humorous account of his conversion. The event that turned the tide was an exhibition by John Grimek, a two-time Mr. America and former member of the U.S. Olympic weightlifting team, and John Davis, the then-current national and world (and soon to be Olympic) weightlifting champion. Karpovich was astounded by the speed, coordination and flexibility of these two massively-muscled athletes.

To set the scene, Dr. Karpovich explained that as a boy he had been told "that a professional wrestler or strongman could not reach to scratch between his shoulder blades and had to pay a penny to some boy to do this scratching." The exhibition gave the good doctor the opportunity to check it out for himself.

Here's how he told the story on himself: "One day, Bob Hoffman [publisher of *Strength & Health* and coach of the then-world champion U.S. weightlifting team] visited Springfield College to give a lecture and demonstrate weight lifting. He brought along John Grimek and John Davis. The lecture and demonstration were very impressive. During the question period, the opportunity arose to test the legend. Very sweetly, Dr. Karpovich said, addressing Mr. Hoffman, 'will you please ask Mr. Grimek to scratch his back between the shoulder blades?' There was silence. Hoffman looked at Grimek, Grimek looked at Hoffman. Then they and everyone else looked at Dr. Karpovich.

"Said Hoffman, 'And why do you want Grimek to scratch his back?'

"'Because I have been told that weight lifters are so muscle-bound that they cannot scratch their backs.'

"'Well, John,' said Hoffman, ad-

> **Grimek gave Dr. Karpovich "a display of gymnastics and flexibility that astounded him. He did full splits, backbends, handstands, and bent forward to place his elbows close to the floor without bending his knees."**

dressing Grimek, 'oblige the doctor and scratch your back.' And Grimek did, first with one hand, then the other. He scratched from above the shoulder and then below. Davis did the same. The audience roared with laughter at the expense of Dr. Karpovich.

"Both men had huge muscles and, therefore, *should have been* muscle-bound. But they were like the bumblebee who flies, although expert aviation engineers have proved mathematically that a bumblebee cannot fly. This anecdote only illustrates how strongly we may cling to our prejudices and pass on unfounded 'information.'"

Expanding on the incident in *Iron Game History*, Jim Murray said Grimek did a lot more than scratch his back; he gave Dr.

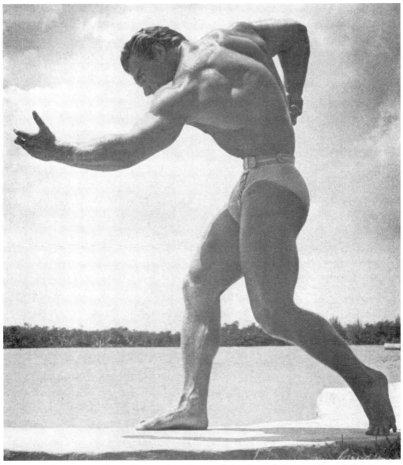

This is John Grimek at about the time of the breakthrough exhibition at Springfield College. You can see why Dr. Karpovich was impressed. *Photo courtesy of Judge Dan Sawyer.*

Karpovich "a display of gymnastics and flexibility that astounded him. Grimek showed full splits, backbends, handstands, and bent forward to place his elbows close to the floor without bending his knees. Needless to say, Dr. Karpovich was impressed."

That unforgettable incident prompted Dr. Karpovich to undertake an experiment to test whether the then-commonly-held belief that weight trainers are slow might also be wrong.

He decided to study speed of arm movement, because arm development was an area where weight trainers clearly stand out from other athletes. He devised a machine that measured the speed with which a subject could turn a handle in front of his chest, using these outsized muscles.

The study involved 600 men, divided equally between men who had never trained with weights (sedentary liberal arts students and vigorous physical education students) and experienced weight lifters and bodybuilders. Much to the doctor's surprise, the weight trainers were faster by a statistically significant margin than the non-lifters; the P.E. students were second and the sedentary students were slowest.

After having debunked the musclebound myth to his complete satisfaction, Dr. Karpovich became an advocate of weight training and remained so for the rest of his life. Calling Dr. Karpovich "weightlifting's non-lifting Patron Saint," Murray freely acknowledges that having him as co-author made their book acceptable to physical educators and coaches—it was used as a textbook for many years—and "paved the way for the present belief that strength training is essential for success in just about every sport."

Returning to the present, it's important to note that it wasn't curls and other isolation exercises that made John Grimek the marvelous athletic specimen that so impressed Dr. Karpovich. That's not to say that Grimek didn't do his share of curls and pumping exercises. He certainly did. But he also did athletic-type lifts that require acceleration, speed, strength, flexibility and intense mental concentration.

> **It was a combination of athletic-type lifts and conventional bodybuilding training that made Grimek the most famous bodybuilder of his time.**

On the occasion of John's retirement from the York Barbell Company in 1985, Bob Hoffman (the same Bob Hoffman who took Grimek and John Davis to Springfield College) wrote an editorial tribute in *Strength & Health*, which included the following comments about Grimek's training:

"When John began training, the popular philosophy stressed the development of an all-around athlete, skilled in a variety of areas.

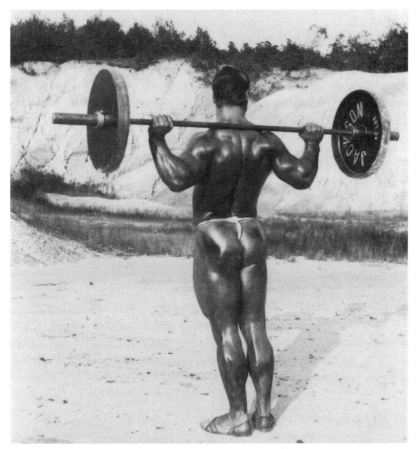

This early photo of John Grimek (*courtesy of the Todd-McLean Collection*) shows the massive hips, thighs and lower back he developed with the aid of athletic-type strength training.

"Hence, it was common for trainees of the time to include the Olympic lifts in their workouts for the acquisition of speed and explosive strength, the slower brute-strength-promoting lifts such as the Squat and Deadlift, standard muscle pumping movements, running and jumping drills, and even strongman stunts.

"John followed this scheme and... became terrifically proficient in just about every category... He was an international caliber Olympic lifter before he became the personna of bodybuilding. In fact, ...he was one of the first to apply the squat style of lifting to the Snatch and [Clean & Jerk]."

So, it was a combination of athletic-type lifts and conventional bodybuilding training that made Grimek the most famous bodybuilder of his time. That's also the type of training I'm currently doing.

I realize the current trend is toward specialization; most trainers are bodybuilders or lifters, and never the twain shall meet. And that's fine. I believe a person should do what provides him or her with the most enjoyment and satisfaction. But for those interested in combining the two types of training, one of the routines in the next chapter includes the Power Snatch and Power Clean as optional exercises. We'll discuss these "quick" lifts when we get to those routines.

Now let's move on to some impressive new information about in high-intensity aerobic training. Those of you who have always tried to stay in the so-called "fat burn" zone to maximize fat loss will be especially interested in this section.

Forget the Fat-Burn Zone

Like high-set bodybuilding, low-intensity endurance exercise has never appealed to me. I'm just not suited for it. As you'll recall, the only event I lost in the high school fitness competition was the 300-yd shuttle run. When I wrestled in high school, I was way back in the pack when the team ran laps after practice. And, as you might imagine, I hated running at Lackland Air Force Base during basic training. Pretty clearly, I'm built more for strength than endurance training.

My guess is that's true for most people who gravitate towards lifting and bodybuilding. You're not likely to see many strength athletes winning marathons, or vice versa. Big strong muscles are just not compatible with prolonged endurance events. If you want to get technical, endurance athletes usually have a preponderance of fatigue-resistant, slow-twitch muscle fibers and weight lifters a preponderance of quick-to-tire, fast-twitch fibers.

This creates a problem for weight trainers who want to use aerobic exercise for fat loss. As explained in *Ripped 3* and *Lean For Life*, endurance exercise can work against gains in strength and muscle size. The traditional answer to this dilemma has been to do very mild cardiovascular training, which was thought to burn calories and fat without interfering with strength and muscle mass.

I've sensed for a some time that this was not the best solution. As those who have read *Ripped* know, the only aerobic exercise I did while training for the Past-40 Mr. America and Mr. U.S.A. competitions was a very hard bike ride once a week.

Refining my approach, in *Ripped 3* I recommended "a variety of relatively short and infrequent aerobic sessions interspersed with explosive muscular effort." In *Lean For Life*, published a few years later, I emphasized intensity even more. I reduced the frequency of aerobic sessions to two times a week—in *Ripped 3*, I recommended up to four—and substantially increased the intensity.

So, I've long believed in brief and infrequent high-intensity aerobics. As my wife will tell you, I'm frequently ahead of the crowd. She tells people to buy the same stocks I do, but wait two years. That's how it's been with high-intensity aerobics. I had it basically correct, but there was a dearth of scientific support for my view. Well, some researchers have finally come to my rescue. They have shown that high-intensity aerobics is best for both fitness and fat loss—especially for strength athletes.

Low-intensity aerobic activity does not necessarily lead to a greater expenditure of calories from fat.

I knew I was on the right track when I perused my copy of *Physiology of Sport and Exercise*, the beautifully designed textbook by Professors Jack H. Wilmore (University of Texas at Austin) and David L. Costill (Ball State University, Muncie, Indiana) published by Human Kinetics in 1994. There it was in black and white: "Low-intensity aerobic activity does not necessarily lead to a greater expenditure of calories from fat. More importantly, the total caloric expenditure for a given period of time is much less when compared with high-intensity activity." In effect, Wilmore and Costill, long revered by runners for their expertise in the field of aerobic exercise, said the often heard recommendation to keep exercise intensity low in order to maximize the loss of body fat—advice to stay in the fat-burn zone—is wrong. Let's say that again because it's important: Any advice to stay in the fat burn zone when doing aerobic exercise so you will burn more fat is wrong.

To illustrate the fat-burn fallacy, they give the example of a 23-year-old woman who exercised for 30 minutes at 50% of her VO_2max on one day, and for 30 minutes at 75% on another. The total calories from fat were the same—in both sessions she burned 110 calories from fat. More importantly, however, in the higher intensity workout she expended about 50 percent more calories for the same time period, 220 total calories for the 50% intensity workout and 332 for the 75% session.

For an average 40-year-old male, the calories from fat would be about 145 in both sessions, but the total calories burned during the higher intensity workout would be 435 compared to only 290 in the low-intensity session, again 50 percent more. That's a big difference and over time the higher-intensity sessions will produce far more fat loss.

A short time later, I had the opportunity to discuss this point

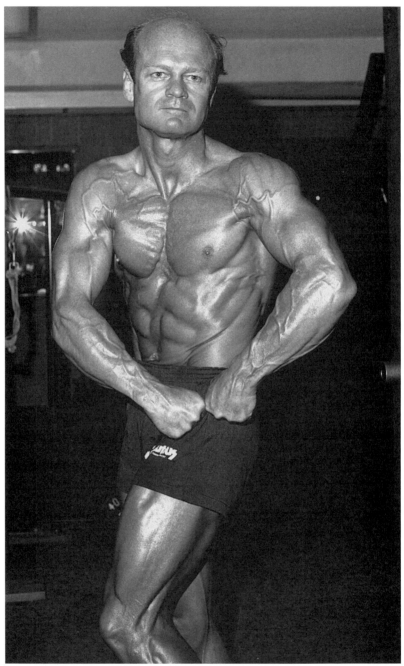

This photo appears on the cover of *Ripped*, my first book. *It was taken by Bill Reynolds* on the day after I won the "Most Muscular Man" award at the Past-40 Mr. USA. I was doing high-intensity aerobics even then, a very hard bike ride once a week.

with Dr. Robert Robergs, director of the Center for Exercise at the University of New Mexico and co-author of *Exercise Physiology: Exercise Performance and Clinical Applications* (Mosby, 1997). Interestingly, Dr. Robergs studied under Costill at Ball State University. Supporting his mentor's pronouncement, Robergs said, "You can't convert a relative contribution to an absolute value; it's the total amount of calories [burned] that's most important."

"There's another issue too," Robergs added, which makes the intensity of the workout important for fat loss. A more intense approach, he explained, "is more conducive to improving the muscle's ability to use fat." The more fit you become, the more likely you are to use fat as fuel. "When you become more fit you are better able to metabolize fat for any given activity you do," Robergs stressed. In other words, you not only burn more calories during workouts, you train your body to burn fat 24 hours a day.

> **You don't stop burning fat when exercise intensity goes above the so called fat-burn zone, as many people have been led to believe. You still burn the same amount of fat, but you burn more calories and—this is very important—you challenge the body to adapt and burn fat more readily.**

That's the bottom line. You don't stop burning fat when exercise intensity goes above the so called fat-burn zone, as many people have been led to believe. You still burn the same amount of fat, but you burn more calories and—this is very important—you challenge the body to adapt and burn fat more readily. It's important to fix the information in this paragraph in your mind as it is the key to maximum fat reduction in aerobic exercise.

Even *Runner's World* magazine agrees with this general proposition. In the July 1998 issue, long-time senior writer Hal Higdon wrote: "High-intensity training can help with weight loss." He added parenthetically, "A half-dozen short bursts of 60 to 90 seconds will do the job." (High-intensity interval training is the topic discussed in the next section.)

What's more, my friend Dr. Richard A. Winett, editor and publisher of the excellent *Master Trainer* newsletter (for a sample copy, send $1 to Suite 221, Memorial Building, 610 N. Main St., Blacksburg, VA 24060-3349), called my attention to cutting-edge research which helps to fill in the details on why high-intensity aerobic exercise is so effective for both fitness and fat loss.

Because of their importance we are going to review two key studies from Japan and Canada. The Japanese research we first review focuses on the effectiveness of high-intensity aerobics for fitness. Short, hard aerobic exercise produced amazing results compared to moderate intensity exercise—in a fraction of the time. The second study, from Canada, shows the results of high-intensity aerobics on fat loss.

Intervals for Fitness

Dr. Izumi Tabata and his colleagues at the National Institute of Fitness and Sports in Tokyo compared the effects of moderate-intensity endurance training and high-intensity interval training on VO_2max (aerobic capacity) and anaerobic capacity. (In general terms, one's ability to continue exercising in the face of rising oxygen debt and lactic acid buildup is called anaerobic capacity.) Their findings are reported in *Medicine and Science in Sports and Exercise*, volume 28, pages 1327-1330 (1996).

Interestingly, the high-intensity protocol had been used by major members of the Japanese national speed skating team for several years; it's a real-world training plan. You'll see, however, that the protocol is unique among aerobic training programs for its intensity and brevity. The moderate-intensity program, on the other hand, is anything but unique. It's the same steady-state aerobic training done by many (perhaps most) fitness enthusiasts.

The moderate-intensity group exercised on stationary bicycles five days per week, for six weeks, at 70% of VO_2max, for 60 minutes each session. (Sound familiar?)

The high-intensity group followed a very unusual—and very short—interval training program five days a week. After a 10-minute warm-up, they did seven to eight sets of 20 seconds at 170% of $V0_2$max, with a 10 second rest period between each bout. The protocol was altered one day per week. On that day, the students exercised for 30 minutes at 70% of their aerobic capacity before doing 4 sets of 20 second intervals at 170%. The first 4 sessions were to exhaustion, but the altered session was not.

Note the duration of the two protocols: one hour compared to about four-minutes!

Most people would probably predict that the longer workout was more effective. They'd be wrong.

The 60-minute moderate-intensity protocol produced a respectable increase in $V0_2$max of 10 percent, but had no effect on anaerobic capacity. The 4-minute program of high-intensity intervals improved $V0_2$max by 14 percent. Anaerobic capacity increased by a whopping 28 percent.

If this sounds remarkable, it is. But not because the brief interval program increased anaerobic capacity and the 60-minute program did not. That was to be expected, because the intensity of the first protocol (70% of VO_2max) did not stress anaerobic capacity; it was not intense enough to produce an oxygen debt or lactic acid buildup. Therefore, it was predictable that anaerobic capacity would be unchanged. On the other hand, the high-intensity group exercised to exhaustion; their anaerobic capacity was taxed to the max. As the researchers explained: "For most properties the more demanding the training is the greater the improvement in the property." That, of course, is the well-known specificity principle.

The surprise was the increase in VO_2max. In an e-mail response to Dick Winett, Dr. Tabata said, "The fact is that the rate of increase in VO_2max [14 percent for the high-intensity protocol—in only 6 weeks] is one of the highest ever reported in exercise science."

> "The 20-second intervals, with 10-second rest periods, overload both aerobic and anaerobic capacity maximally—with the predictable result that both systems benefit. As the original research report stated: "[It] may be one of the best possible training protocols..."

The improvement is all the more remarkable, because the student participants were members of varsity table tennis, baseball, basketball, soccer and swimming teams. They already had relatively high aerobic capacities.

Moreover, the 4-minute training program of very hard 20-second repeats, in the words of the peer-reviewed research report, "may be optimal with respect to improving both the aerobic and the anaerobic energy release systems."

In short, like Goldilock's porridge, it seems that Dr. Tabata and his colleagues—with an assist from the Japanese speed skaters—have come upon an interval program that is "just right." As was shown in a follow-up study (*Medicine and Science in Sports and Exercise* (1997) 29, 390-395), the 20-second intervals, with 10-second rest periods, overload both aerobic and anaerobic capacity maximally—with the predictable result that both systems benefit. As the original research report stated: "[It] may be one of the best possible training protocols..."

That's why I've incorporated the Tabata protocol in my own training and why you'll find it in the routines in the next chapter. Of course, this type of training should only be undertaken by those in good condition. As you will see in the exercise section, Dr. Tabata specifically includes a warning to this effect.

Now, let's move on to the Canadian study which demonstrates the efficacy of high-intensity intervals for fat loss.

Intervals for Fat Loss

Like Drs. Wilmore and Costill, Angelo Tremblay, Ph.D., and his colleagues at Laval University in Canada challenged the common belief among health professionals (see footnote below) that low-intensity, long-duration exercise is the best program for fat loss. They compared the impact of moderate-intensity aerobic exercise and high-intensity intervals on fat loss. (*Metabolism* (1994) Volume 43, pp 814-818)

The Canadian scientists divided inactive adults into two groups. One group, the endurance training group (ET), did uninterrupted cycling for 30–45 minutes, 4 or 5 times a week, for 20 weeks. The intensity was greater than usually prescribed for weight or fat loss. It began at 60 percent of heart rate reserve and progressed to 85 percent. For a 30-year-old, this would mean starting at a heart rate of about 136 and progressing to roughly 170.

The other group did a 15-week program primarily made up of high-intensity interval training (HIIT). Much like the ET group, they began with 30 minutes of continuous cycling at 70 percent of heart rate reserve—remember they were not accustomed to exercise—but soon progressed to intervals. The HIIT group did 10 to 15 short (15 seconds progressing to 30 seconds) or 4 to 5 long (60 seconds progressing to 90 seconds) intervals, separated by relatively long recovery periods. The rest intervals were long enough to allow heart rate to drop to 120-130 beats per minute. The intensity of the short intervals was initially fixed at 60 percent of each subject's maximal work output for 10 seconds; and the intensity of the long intervals corresponded to 70 percent of individual maximum work output in 90 seconds. Intensity for both long and short intervals was increased 5 percent every three weeks. In short, these were hard intervals.

> In the final analysis, the HIIT group got nine times more fat loss benefit for every calorie burned exercising.

Significantly, the total energy cost of the ET program was substantially greater than the HIIT program. The researchers calculated that the ET group burned more than twice as many calories while exercising than the HIIT group. But—surprise, surprise—skinfold measurements showed that the HIIT group

---

Citing 28 references to support their position, the American College of Sports Medicine recommends 20 to 60 minutes of continuous aerobic activity. But Dr. Ralph Carpinelli, who teaches the neuromuscular aspects of strength training at Adelphi University (NY), reviewed all 28 references and reported in *Master Trainer* (August 1998) that only three studies actually support the claim that duration is the major stimulus for adapation.

lost more subcutaneous fat. "Moreover," reported the researchers, "when the difference in the total energy cost of the program was taken into account…, the subcutaneous fat loss was *ninefold greater* in the HIIT group than in the ET program." In the final analysis, the HIIT group got nine times more fat loss benefit for every calorie burned exercising.

How is that possible?

Dr. Tremblay's group took muscle biopsies and measured muscle enzyme activity to determine why high-intensity intervals produced so much more fat loss. I'll spare you the details (they're quite technical and hard to decipher) but here's the bottom line: "[Metabolic adaptation resulting from HIIT] may lead to a better lipid [fat] utilization in the post exercise state and this contributes to a greater energy and lipid deficit." In other words, compared to moderate-intensity continuous endurance exercise, high-intensity intermittent exercise causes more calories and fat to be burned *following* the workout. Citing animal studies, they also said it may be that appetite is suppressed more following intense intervals. (Neither group was placed on a diet.) Both explanations have found additional support.

The August 1998 *Master Trainer* reported: "[Other research] indicates that while increasing the duration of low intensity exercise results in linear increases in total energy expended during recovery, increases in intensity of exercise appear to *exponentially* increase energy expended during recovery." That means increasing intensity stirs up the system (heart rate, breathing, oxygen debt, lactic acid buildup and muscle cell damage, for example) by a substantially greater order of magnitude—exactly how much is unknown—than extending duration to the same degree. Therefore, it takes more energy, including that provided by fat metabolism, to restore the body to normal status.

Regarding the second rationale given by the Tremblay group, I know that I'm not hungry after an intense aerobic session; I eat my normal meal anyway, of course. A follow-up study by Imbeault, Saint-Pierre, Almeras and Tremblay (*British Journal of Nutrition* (1997) 77, 511-521) suggests that I'm not atypical.

This study measured perceived hunger and fullness, and calorie consumption after three conditions: quiet reading, low-intensity exercise on a treadmill (35% of VO_2max) and high-intensity exercise on a treadmill (75% VO_2max). Somewhat surprisingly, the subjects reported the same hunger and fullness, and ate the same number of calories after all three conditions. However—this is the key point—the subjects doing high-intensity exercise consumed fewer calories in relation to the full energy cost during and after exercise.

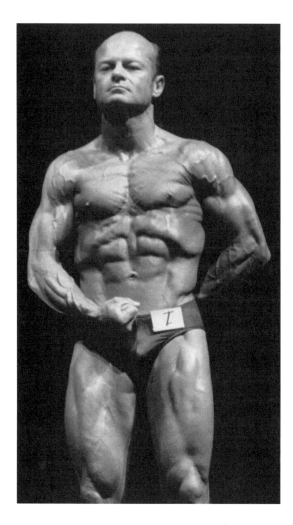

High intensity aerobics helped me achieve this degree of leanness on stage at the Past-40 Mr. USA. *Photo by Ken Sprague.*

Again, the main determinant was the post-exercise metabolic cost. (The study design made the energy cost of the active exercise the same.) Those doing high-intensity exercise burned more calories after the exercise session—but consumed the same number of calories as those who read quietly or did low-intensity exercise. The researchers concluded: "...Increased exercise intensity allows satiety with reduced energy intake relative to energy expenditure."

So, the animal studies cited in the earlier Tremblay report were predictive of human behavior. When I burn more calories doing high-intensity intervals—but eat the same as always—I come out ahead from the fat loss standpoint.

In summary, high-intensity aerobic exercise—especially the short and long intervals in the original Tremblay study—burns more calories per minute of exercise and more calories—and fat—

during recovery. What's more, even though it burns more total calories, high-intensity aerobics doesn't seem to increase appetite more than equal amounts of low-intensity aerobics. Finally, and perhaps most importantly, high-intensity intervals appear to cause metabolic changes which improve the body's ability to burn fat during and after workouts, and around the clock.

You'll find the original Tremblay interval protocols in the new routines as well.

A Barbell Aerobics Strategy

Bond traders sometimes use a "barbell strategy" to diversity their portfolios and reduce risk. For example, at one end of the maturity scale—or barbell—they might buy 30-year Treasury Bonds, which typically pay a high interest rate and carry a high degree of risk, and simultaneously buy lower yielding and less risky short-term bonds at the other end of the yield spectrum—or barbell. This barbell strategy gives them an average yield and risk somewhere in the middle. Don't ask me why they don't just buy intermediate-term bonds, because I'm not sure. What I do know is that I use a similar strategy in my aerobic exercise program. I do a combination of high intensity intervals and low-intensity walking. I completely eliminate the moderate-intensity aerobics that most people do. This works great—and I do know why.

As you already know, our capacity to recover from exercise is a finite quantity; it's limited. As George Sheehan so wisely observed, the proper balance of stress and rest is critical to the success of any exercise program. The problem is compounded, of course, when you combine weights and aerobics.

Naturally, I want the fitness and fat-loss benefits of aerobic exercise; but I don't want to hamper recovery from my weight workouts. In addition, I want the benefits of high-intensity intervals which we've been discussing. High-intensity intervals, of course, require more recovery time. How to enjoy the benefits of high-intensity aerobics, while avoiding the pitfalls? That's the question.

I've tried many ways to accomplish this, and I've almost come full-circle in the process of discovery.

As mentioned, when I began training for the Past-40 Mr.

What's more, even though it burns more total calories, high-intensity aerobics doesn't seem to increase appetite more than equal amounts of low-intensity aerobics. Finally, and perhaps most importantly, high-intensity intervals appear to cause metabolic changes which improve the body's ability to burn fat during and after workouts, and around the clock.

America contest and first began thinking seriously about the best way to combine weights and aerobics, I did only one aerobics session per week, a hard bike ride of about 20 miles. Since then, I've tried up to 4 aerobics sessions a week. Through trial and error, I've come to the conclusion that I had it almost right at the outset. One hard aerobics session is enough—if combined with frequent walks or some similar activity. In other words, I've adopted a barbell strategy of high- and low-intensity aerobics.

> One hard interval session gives me the desired fitness and fat-burning benefits, without unduly interfering with weight workouts. But it doesn't burn enough calories. Walking solves that problem, and without hurting recovery. In fact, I believe walking aids recovery.

One hard interval session gives me the desired fitness and fat-burning benefits, without unduly interfering with weight workouts. But it doesn't burn enough calories. Walking solves that problem, and without hurting recovery. In fact, I believe walking aids recovery.

We already know that high-intensity intervals make substantial demands on recovery capacity. That's why they cause so many calories to be burned after the workout. So, let's focus on the advantages of walking.

A careful reading of an article on fat burn during exercise in *The Physician And Sportsmedicine* (Sept 1998) reveals my reason for walking. The author, John A. Hawley, Ph.D., starts with a key point: "The relative contributions of fat and carbohydrate vary with intensity." That's important to understand, because high-intensity aerobics burns carbohydrate (glycogen) and fat stored in the muscles. This, of course, is part of the process of muscle breakdown—and impedes recovery.

Comfortable walking is the answer to the recovery problem. "Low intensity activities such as walking strongly stimulate lipolysis [fat burn] from peripheral adipocytes [fat deposits], while intramuscular triglycerides [fat] contribute little or nothing to total energy expenditure," Dr. Hawley explains. "Carbohydrate needs are met predominately by circulating blood glucose, with little or no muscle glycogen breakdown."

That says it all. Walking at a comfortable pace burns fat from outlying deposits—love handle fat, for example—as differentiated from intermuscular fat. The small amount of energy that comes from carbohydrates is supplied by blood sugar, and not by glucose stored in the muscles. That's ideal, of course, for an athlete who wants to burn fat without disturbing ongoing recovery inside the muscles.

92

The icing on the cake is that walking actually aids recovery. It stimulates circulation, bringing the building blocks of recovery to the muscles and carrying away the waste products generated by high-intensity exercise.

Needless to say, the new routines are laced with comfortable walking. I don't recommend fast or "speed" walking, because I don't want to turn walking into a workout. That would defeat the purpose. Fast walking is good exercise, but it depletes the small amount of fat and carbohydrate stored in the muscles. That delays recovery. Our walking is to burn fat located in undesirable areas—and speed recovery.

As I promised at the start, we've covered a lot of exciting, new material in this chapter. Now, let's put the information to work in the new routines.

"Exactly contrary to the generally-practiced rule, advanced trainees should actually train less than they did earlier—but much harder."

—Arthur Jones
Nautilus Training Principles
Bulletin No. 2

"I predict that periodization, which in essence is nothing more than the careful planning of a long-term program, will eventually become more popular with bodybuilders because a lot of them are fed up at not making any progress."

—Charles Poliquin
The Poliquin Principles

CHAPTER FIVE

The New Routines

New Challenges

These routines, which incorporate the training concepts we've been discussing, present exciting new ways to challenge yourself. They are not intended to replace or eclipse the routines in the earlier books, but rather to provide new options to keep your training fresh and interesting.

> **The second routine melds the two types of training to build maximum muscle size—and strength—by promoting both energy substrate storage and enlargement of the contractile fibers.**

As I said before, there is no single "best way" to train, certainly not for everyone in every circumstance. There are many productive ways to train. To keep making progress—especially if you've been training for some time—you have to keep changing your workout plan. New challenges prod your body into further rounds of adaptation.

Remember the virtuous circle we talked about in the last chapter? Training satisfaction comes from progress, and it's training satisfaction that motivates you to keep striving—and progressing. These routines are designed to keep the cycle going. They keep you training and gaining. Enjoy.

About the New Routines

There are three new weight training routines, each with a different focus. The first routine is "the entry-level routine." It focuses on a group I haven't emphasized before: beginners or people who have been away from training for an extended period of time. It's been a long time since I was a beginner, but I realize that entry-level bodybuilders have special needs. Even if you are not a beginner, I urge you to peruse the first routine, because it introduces concepts which are also part of the other routines.

The second routine is "the mass and strength routine." Following thorough on an idea put forth in the last chapter, it combines volume training and high-intensity training in an effort to produce the best of both worlds. It melds the two types of training to build maximum muscle size—and strength—by promoting both energy substrate storage and enlargement of the contractile fibers. This is a new concept to me, and I believe it has exciting possibilities.

The final routine is my current training program. It includes athletic-type lifts such as the Power Snatch and Power Clean, which require strength, speed and coordination. These are the lifts which contributed so much to John Grimek's magnificent physique. I realize, however,

> **The Tabata and Tremblay interval protocols are perfect for bodybuilders and strength athletes.**

that some will be reluctant to do the quick lifts, so I have made them optional. The routine can be done quite effectively without the Snatch and Clean, because the workouts include other multi-joint exercises that involve the major muscles of the body working together.

For those who have been writing, calling and e-mailing for more details, the high-intensity aerobic protocols discussed in the last chapter are also a major part of the final routine. The Tabata and Tremblay interval protocols offer a new way to burn fat and build aerobic fitness. Plus, they are wonderfully challenging and fun. I believe they are perfect for bodybuilders and strength athletes.

Perhaps the most controversial aspect of the third and final routine is that the weight and aerobics sessions are performed only once a week. I'll explain why that works when we get to the details of the routine.

All three routines include planned change, which is the essence of periodization, the concept we discussed earlier. Training cycles are divided into phases of varying length. Volume is generally high at the beginning and decreases from phase to phase; intensity, on the other hand, begins relatively low and peaks in the final phase. There is a rhythm to the training cycles; the volume and intensity ebb and flow. In general, you push for a while, back off, and then push again.

> **Perhaps the most controversial aspect of the third and final routine is that the weight and aerobics sessions are performed only once a week.**

As I said earlier, periodization is a wonderful and satisfying way to train. Done properly, you almost never hit a sticking point. Your performance escalates from phase to phase and you end each cycle a little bigger, stronger and fitter than before. Instead of frustration, you experience one success after another. And that keeps you motivated. Success breeds success.

The first two routines, the entry-level and the mass and strength routines, include more sets than the workouts in my earlier books. This is to take advantage of the benefits of volume training discussed in the last chapter. The third routine, my current routine, however, sticks for the most part to the one-set-after-warmup philosophy. When we get to the final routine, I'll tell you about new research which confirms the value of time-efficient, one-set training.

> **I thought it was time to emphasize the efficiency and utility of training the whole body in one workout.**

Finally, in another departure from my earlier books, the workouts in all three routines cover the whole body. That's not meant to denigrate split routines, where body parts are trained on different days. Split routines are ideal in many circumstances, but I thought it was time to emphasize the efficiency and utility of training the whole body in one workout.

Before we move on to the first routine, I want to clarify a presentation point that may cause confusion. Intensity in the weight routines is expressed as a percentage. The percentage relates to your maximum for the number of repetitions to be performed. For example, if 12 repetitions with 100 pounds is your limit, then 100 pounds would be 100% of your 12-repetition maximum, and 85 pounds would be 85% of your 12-rep maximum.

Note that this is different than some other books which express intensity as a percentage of one-repetition maximum (1RM). Using 1RM, of course, requires that you determine how much weight you can lift for one repetition in each exercise. I believe that's confusing, unnecessary and in some cases dangerous. So again, all percentage figures in this book relate to the number of reps called for in the routine. As I'll remind you in each routine, 50/12-2 means two sets of 12 reps with 50% of your 12-rep maximum. Put another way using a second example, 85/10-3 means 85% of your 10-rep max, 10 reps, 3 sets.

The actual weight used will, of course, be unique to you. You'll have to experiment a little, particularly on new exercises and repetition ranges, but you'll soon find your current maximum poundages.

It's important to keep in mind that your maximum will keep changing. As you continue to lift, you'll become stronger and be able to lift more weight in each exercise. That's what training is all about, overloading your muscles and getting bigger and stronger. You simply adjust your training poundages as you progress. The percentage figures will always refer to your current max for the number of reps called for in the training plan.

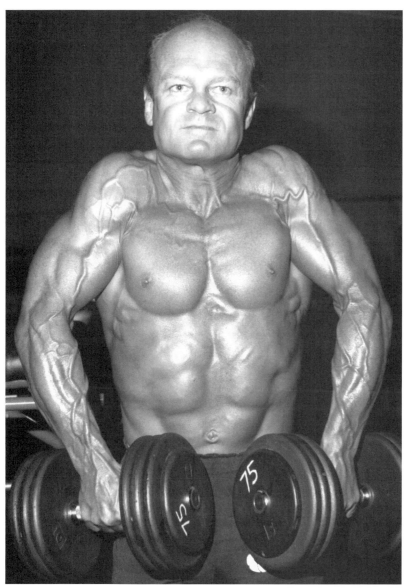

As you continue to lift, you'll become stronger and be able to lift more weight in each exercise. That's what training is all about, overloading your muscles and getting bigger and stronger. *Photo by Bill Reynolds.*

The Entry-Level Routine

My book *Lean For Life* does not include an entry-level routine, but it does contain an excellent section called "Help For Beginners," which I recommend to anyone embarking on a weight training program for the first time. It contains a list of information sources (most of which are available from Ripped Enterprises), including *Biomarkers*, a book by William Evans, Ph.D. and Irwin H. Rosenberg, M.D., both professors of nutrition and medicine.

I want to mention *Biomarkers* again, because it includes a 16-week catch-up program for unfit individuals who may not be ready to start lifting barbells and dumbbells right away. The authors start you out walking on day one and gradually ease you into a simple resistance program that can be done at home using chairs, stools and other basic household items. *Biomarkers* also has an excellent chapter on basic exercise concepts, including strength-building fundamentals and safety guidelines.

Aerobic exercise and diet are important, but strength training is pivotal if you want to stay young longer.

Even if you are fit enough to begin a full-blown weight workout—check with your doctor if you have any doubts whatsoever about your physical status, or in any event if you're over 35 and have not been exercising regularly—you should read *Biomarkers* for the ground-breaking research information it provides. This landmark book presents dramatic evidence that strength training may be even more important than aerobics in retarding the aging process.

Evans and Rosenberg say the two most important biomarkers—signposts of vitality that indicate one's physiological age—are muscle mass and strength. They're the lead dominoes, so to speak.

When your muscle mass and strength start to topple, the other indications of aging soon make their appearance. Preserve your muscular strength, however, and the rest of you will hold up as well. Aerobic exercise and diet are important, but strength training, according to Evans and Rosenberg, is pivotal if you want to stay young longer.

Another book referred to in *Lean For Life* is *Keys To The Inner Universe* by bodybuilding legend Bill Pearl. *Keys* is an encyclopedia of bodybuilding. It weighs in at five pounds, contains more than 600 pages, and has the most complete list of weight training exercises ever assembled. Every piece of equipment and every exercise imaginable is included with drawings and explanatory text. I'll give you a few tips on exercise performance, but if you need more instruction Pearl's book is the place to go (it's available from Ripped Enterprises). A beginner might also find it worthwhile to sign up at a local fitness center for a month or two of basic weight training instruction, or perhaps hire a personal trainer to help you with the performance of the basic exercises included in this routine. Needless to say, you'll find books in any large bookstore on basic weight training.

If you're over 50 and want to begin weight training, an excellent book to get you started properly is *Strength Training Past 50* by Wayne L. Westcott and Thomas R. Baechle (Human Kinetics, 1998). Westcott and Baechele are world-renowned experts and well-qualified to help over-50 beginners. (This book is also available from Ripped Enterprises.)

With those preliminaries out of the way, it's time to get down to the business of preparing your body for heavy weight training. That's the purpose of the entry-level routine.

Preparing Your Body

Some degree of soreness is practically unavoidable at the beginning of any new weight training program. That's true even if you've been training for a long time, like I have. I welcome — and expect — soreness when I do an exercise I haven't done for a while or begin a new workout plan. This type of soreness is called "delayed onset muscle soreness," because it doesn't really hit you until a day or two later.

DOMS is completely natural. Your body is simply telling you it has been subjected to a new stress. That's good. That's overload, which you'll remember is the basic principle — the driving force — of weight training. Progressive overload builds muscle.

If you want to get technical, the aches, pains and stiffness you feel are caused by microscopic tears in your muscle cells. The tears, in turn, cause inflammation and swelling, which hurts. As you'll remember from our discussion of the muscle cell damage or wound healing theory of recovery, inflammation is part of the process by which our muscles adapt to weight training. Recall also that the degree of damage depends on the intensity of the exercise. In Dave Staplin's words, "The higher the intensity, the greater the damage." And, we should add, the greater the soreness.

That's why it's important to ease into any new exercise program. If you start off too vigorously, the result can be almost crippling soreness. The worst kind of soreness involves not only the muscles but also the ligaments and tendons that support the joints and attach muscles to bones. If you don't take it easy at the start, these supporting structures can complain to the extent that you won't be able to straighten your arms or stand up straight. The muscles usually adjust to weight training in a few weeks, but the tendons and ligaments need more time, probably because they are more rigid and have less circulation than muscle tissue.

That's a long winded way of explaining why this routine starts you out lifting at only half power. If you can lift 100 pounds for 12 reps, you are asked to restrict yourself to only 50 pounds in the first week. Please resist the temptation to lift more. This entry-level routine lasts 12 weeks. The challenging stuff will come soon enough; in week 12, you'll be using 85% of your 12-rep maximum. That means the last set will be plenty hard.

> **Beginners and out-of-shape individuals need volume more than intensity to condition their bodies to cope with the heavier loads to come.**

Ease into weight training as suggested here and your body—especially your tendons and ligaments—will thank you for being patient. You'll avoid injury and will not get overly sore. What's more, you'll enjoy the process of preparing your body to benefit from more demanding workouts.

The Rhythm of the Routine Is Important

Unlike most of my routines, the amount of training, or volume, stays about the same for all 12 weeks. Two or three sets of 12 reps are recommended for each exercise. That's because beginners and out-of-shape individuals need volume more than intensity to condition their bodies to cope with the heavier loads to come. That's also why this routine suggests training your whole body three times a week.

As already indicated, the poundages gradually increase, but not in a straight line. You push for a while, back off to give your body time to adjust, and then you push again. The intensity changes every week.

The rhythm of the routine is important. The occasional retreats are characteristic of most periodization plans. They give the body a reprieve to allow it to renew itself in preparation for the next surge forward. This ebb and flow is what keeps you gaining month after month and year after year.

Only Six Exercises

There are two workouts in the entry-level routine, A and B. Each workout consists of only six exercises and lasts six weeks.

102

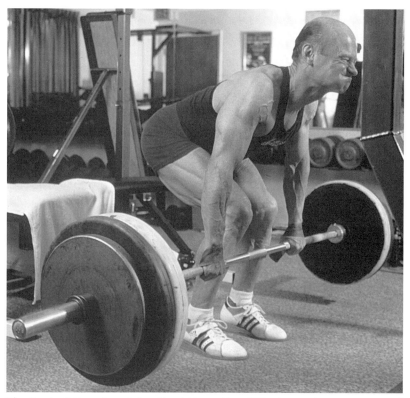

The Barbell Squat and the Bent-Knee Deadlift, shown here, are two of my favorite exercises. I almost always include them in my workouts. *Photo by Pat Berrett*

Having only six exercises keeps the sessions manageable; you should be able to complete the workouts in under an hour, including warm-up and cooldown (which we'll get to shortly). The actual length will depend on how long you rest between sets and exercises. Take as long as you need; don't rush, but don't let your muscles get cold. Forty-five minutes to an hour is about the ideal length for a training session. Go longer and you tend to lose your drive and enthusiasm.

The workouts are made up of basic exercises that work several muscle groups together. The calf raise is the only single-joint exercise. The other exercises involve several joints, which means that many muscles are working. The best examples are the Bent-Knee Deadlift, in program A, and the Barbell Squat, in program B. These are two of my favorite exercises—I almost always include them in my workouts—because they work the largest and most important muscles of the body. The angle of stress is slightly different, but both the Deadlift and the Squat work the massive muscles of the hips, lower back, frontal thigh and the hamstrings. When these muscles are stimulated, the whole body grows.

There are no arm exercises, no Curls or Triceps Extensions. That's because the Lat Pulldown in workout A and the two rowing movements in workout B stimulate the biceps; and the pressing exercises in both workouts strongly affect the triceps. That demonstrates the advantage of emphasizing the multi-muscle exercises over single-muscle exercises, such as the Arm Curl. They do the job so well that you can train your whole body in a reasonable period of time. As you'll see, multi-muscle exercises predominate in the other routines as well.

A and B Workouts

The A and B workouts complement each other. Take the upper back exercises, for example. The Front Lat Pulldown, in workout A, puts the stress on the upper and outer part of the back, and the Bent-Over Row, in workout B, stresses the middle and lower lats. Together they cover the entire upper back. It works the same for the chest; the Bench Press in A is probably the best overall exercise for the chest—it hits the pectorals squarely—while the Incline Dumbbell Press in the B workout places more stress on the upper pecs. Again, both exercises together train the entire chest.

> A warm-up is necessary to prepare the muscles and joints—and the mind—to train, but it shouldn't be overdone.

I generally stick to exercises, like those included here and in the other two routines, which work a lot of muscles at one time. I've never found that it pays to stray too far from the basic movements. I don't wear myself out trying to isolate individual muscles. I believe most people, especially beginners, would be well advised to follow my lead.

No Aerobic Sessions

Readers of my other books may be surprised that there are no aerobic exercise sessions in this routine or the next routine. That's because both routines include considerably more volume than the routines in my other books. As I said in *Ripped 2*, weight training and aerobics are an ideal combination, "but too much of a good thing causes trouble." Training the whole body with weights three times a week, as called for here, is a lot of exercise, especially for a beginner or someone getting back to training after a long layoff.

Rather than taxing aerobic sessions, which would probably put you over the line into overtraining, I suggest walking for up to an hour on off days. That won't wear you out and, as explained in the last chapter, walking at a comfortable pace aids recovery and burns fat. Plus, it makes you feel good.

Warm-Up and Cool Down

Now, as promised, let's talk about warming up. A warm-up is necessary to prepare the muscles and joints—and the mind—to train, but it shouldn't be overdone. The general rule on warming up is to do enough to prepare yourself for the heavy sets—and no more. Don't waste precious energy and recovery capacity on unnecessary and nonproductive warm-up exercises.

I do a brief general warm-up before starting my weight work-out—nothing fancy, just enough to get the blood flowing all over the body and warm up the joints. I do five or 10 repetitions of each of the following movements:

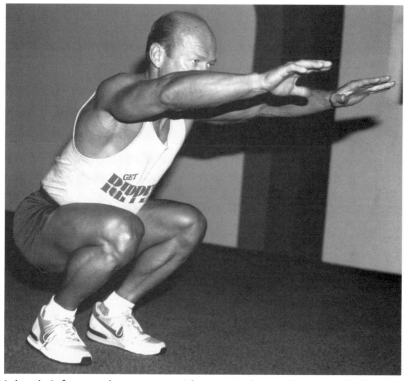

I do a brief general warm-up, without weights, at the start of all training sessions (weights and aerobics). *Photo by Guy Appelman.*

1) curl and extend the arms (rotate palms, up at the top and down on extension) to warm up the elbows and arm muscles;

2) rotate or shrug the shoulders (backward and forward) for the trapezius and upper back;

3) swing the arms to the front and back (like swimming) for the shoulders;

4) high knee lifts (like marching in place) to loosen the hips;

5) bend down and touch the toes (with knees slightly bent) to warm up the lower back and hamstrings;

6) and, finally, squats for the knees (the first few reps can be done with hands on the floor to take some of the weight off the knees initially, and then come upright and continue with full range knee bends).

I recommend that everyone, beginner and advanced alike, do this little routine or something similar at the start of all training sessions (weights and aerobics). It only takes a few minutes and it really helps put you in the mood to train.

I repeat the same movements at the end of each workout. This brings the circulation back to normal. It also helps the muscles get rid of waste products, which speeds recovery and reduces stiffness. This is my cooldown for weight sessions. For hard aerobic sessions, I keep moving until my heart rate drops to about 120, and then I repeat my general warm-up routine.

A specific warm-up is also necessary to prepare for each heavy weight exercise. Again, nothing fancy. Simply do a few reps of the exercise with a light weight. Do only what's necessary to prepare your muscles and joints for a maximum effort.

Both workouts are to be repeated three non-consecutive days each week, Monday, Wednesday and Friday, or Tuesday, Thursday and Saturday, for example.

You'll need more warm-up sets for exercises such as the Squat and Deadlift, where large muscle groups and heavy weights are involved. In general, fewer warm-up sets are necessary for exercises which work the smaller muscles of the upper body. For example, I usually do two or three warm-up sets with progressively heavier weights for Squats or Deadlifts, but only one warm-up set for Curls. There's no need to do a lot of reps. For example, if you plan to do 12 reps in your work sets, 5 reps or less in warm-up sets are plenty.

In this entry-level routine a general warm-up may be all that's necessary, at least at the beginning when the load is only 50 percent of your capacity. Later, when the weights are heavier,

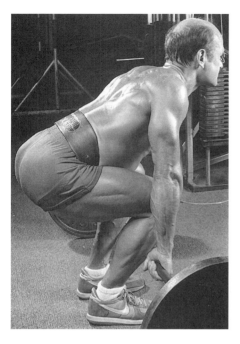

The main thing to remember on the Bent-Knee Deadlift, shown left, and the Barbell Squat, shown below, is to keep your back straight. On the Deadlift, don't attempt to jerk the weight off the floor; pull with the legs, slowly and smoothly, and don't allow your back to round. Keep your back straight as you come erect with the weight. On the Squat, keep your body tight and never go down fast or bounce out of the bottom position; again, don't allow your back to round. On both exercises, control the weight at all times, while lifting and lowering. Many people find that wearing shoes with slightly built-up heels helps them maintain the proper position. **Finally, if you have a bad back or bad knees, consult your physician before doing either movement.** *Photos by Michael Neveux* (top left) and *Guy Appelman*.

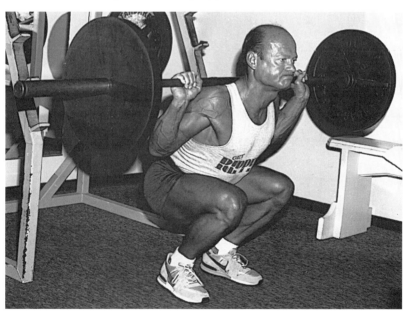

you probably will need a warm-up set or two, especially for the Squat, Deadlift, Row and Bench Press. Just use common sense and do what's necessary. Again, remember the general rule: Do only enough warm-up to prepare adequately for the work sets, no more.

Tips on Exercise Performance

Finally, a few words on exercise performance, and then you'll be ready to start training. If you haven't lifted weights before, I suggest you spend a few days or a week becoming familiar with each exercise, and getting a feel for how much weight you can lift for 12 reps. It's not necessary to actually do a maximum set of 12 reps in each exercise. It's perfectly fine to just experiment a little, and then take your best guess. My only suggestion is that you make it a point to err on the low side. Remember, you will be progressively upping the weights for 12 weeks. If you start too high, you'll not only make yourself unnecessarily sore, you probably won't be able to make all of the increases. You've got plenty of time. You plan to train for years, don't you? Be patient. Go slow. You'll be glad you did.

Explaining how to do standard exercises is beyond the scope of this book, but I would like to give you a few tips on the Deadlift and Squat. Look at the nearby photos of both exercises. Note the position of the lower back. That's the key. On both the Bent-Knee Deadlift and the Barbell Full Squat, keep your body tight throughout the lift, up and down, and maintain the flat back position shown in the photos. *Don't round your back!*

The 12-Week Entry-Level Routine

With that detailed explanation, here's my suggested entry-level routine. It's not written in stone. Many acceptable variations are possible, but I believe this routine provides a good working blueprint for beginners or people returning to weight training after an extended layoff.

As we said, workout A is for weeks 1–6 and workout B is for weeks 7–12. Both workouts are to be repeated three non-consecutive days each week, Monday, Wednesday and Friday, or Tuesday, Thursday and Saturday, for example. Walk on off days (see text). Remember, 50/12-2 means two sets of 12 reps with 50% of your 12-rep maximum. Before you begin, do a brief general warm-up as described above. In addition, warm up for each exercise as necessary (see text). Repeat the general warm-up to cooldown at the end of each session.

Workout A
Week

Exercise	1	2	3	4	5	6
Bent-Knee Deadlift	50/12-2	60/12-2	70/12-2	60/12-3	70/12-3	80/12-3
Standing Calf Raise	same	same	same	same	same	same
Lat Pulldown (front)	same	same	same	same	same	same
Barbell Bench Press	same	same	same	same	same	same
Seated DB Shoulder Press	same	same	same	same	same	same
Abdominal Crunch	10-2	12-2	14-2	12-3	14-3	16-3

(adjust resistance by changing arm position, as necessary)

Workout B
Week

Exercise	7	8	9	10	11	12
Barbell Squart	55/12-2	65/12-2	75/12-2	65/12-3	75/12-3	85/12-3
One-leg Calf Raise w/ DB	same	same	same	same	same	same
Bent-Over Row (DBs)	same	same	same	same	same	same
Incline DB Press	same	same	same	same	same	same
Dumbell Upright Row	same	same	same	same	same	same
Hanging Knee Lift	6-2	8-2	10-2	8-3	10-3	12-3

Now, take a week off. Stay active—walk, bike, do something you enjoy—but take it easy. Give your body a chance to recuperate. Let your enthusiasm return before tackling more demanding workouts, such as those in the next routine, or the routines in *Ripped 3* or *Lean For Life*. If you feel like you need more time to adapt to regular weight training, you can always repeat this routine. If you chose that option, remember that you're stronger now; you'll need to up the poundages some-

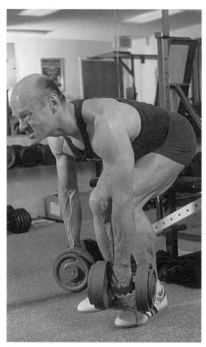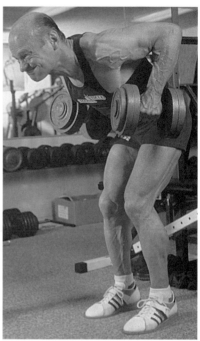

These photos show the start and finish of the Bent-Over Row with dumbbells, which is included in workout B. Like the Squat and Deadlift, it's important to maintain a flat back position, as shown. *Photos by Pat Berrett.*

what to accommodate your new strength level. Don't forget that "progressive" overload is what weight training is all about. Challenge yourself.

Mass and Strength Routine

This is the second routine, which uses periodization to combine volume and high-intensity training. The theories of both types of training are spelled out in the last chapter, so I won't repeat the details here. The bottom line is that fast-paced, volume training builds muscle size mainly by promoting energy substrate storage, and take-your-time, high-intensity training increases the size and strength of the contractile fibers. Melding the two types of training should produce an awesome combination of mass and strength.

Note, however, that the overall volume in this routine is considerably less than Bompa and other proponents of periodization generally recommend. My philosophy is that less is more. Overtraining stymies growth in any system of training.

That's also why there are no formal aerobics workouts in this routine. I suggest you walk at a comfortable pace on off days for up to an hour.

The mass and strength routine consists of three phases, each lasting four weeks:

- Phase one—the volume phase which is my version of volume training
- Phase two—the mixed phase which is a combination of volume and high intensity training
- Phase three—the strength phase which is high intensity training.

The Volume Phase

In the first phase there are two workouts, as in the entry-level program, but here they are done alternately throughout the four weeks. You train three times a week and alternate the workouts every time. This is done to keep the workout sessions reasonably short, but still have enough variation of exercises to work the body completely. For example, one workout includes the One-Arm Dumbbell Row and the other the Lat Pulldown; together, the two exercises work all of the major muscles of the upper back.

Again, we stick to multi-joint or multi-muscle exercises, such as the Squat and Bench Press, that work a lot of muscle all at once. Like spreading the exercises over two workouts, this makes it possible to complete the workouts in one hour or less, and thus maintains drive and enthusiasm.

As explained in the last chapter, the rest intervals between sets are very important when using the volume approach. Bompa says, "The key element in hypertrophy training is the cumulative effect of exhaustion over the total number of sets." With short rest intervals, "the muscles have less time to restore the energy reserves."

Remember that the rest period between sets is very important in volume training; rest 1-2 minutes between sets in this phase

The rationale is basically the same as in the Tabata aerobic interval protocol, which was also discussed in the last chapter. That protocol, as you'll recall, was extremely effective for increasing both aerobic and anaerobic capacity.

Here we are using essentially the same method, but with weights. The idea is to force the muscles to adapt by increasing energy reserves—and muscle size.

111

Rest intervals of 60–120 seconds should do the job. I suggest a range, because you'll need more rest for big muscles such as those in the lower body, and less for small muscles such as the biceps and triceps, with upper back, chest and shoulders falling somewhere in the middle. For example, two minutes is about right for the Squat and Deadlift, 90-seconds for the Bench Press and a minute for Curls. (Some experts recommend shorter rest intervals, but I believe that reduces the stress on the contractile fibers too much; it turns resistance training into aerobics.)

With these short rest intervals, your muscles will fatigue more with each set; you'll be hard put to complete the last few reps of the final set. That's the idea. Incomplete recovery means energy stores are not being fully replenished between sets. If everything—weight, reps and the rest interval—is just right, energy stores will be severely depleted by the end of the last set.

In this routine that won't happen right away, because the poundages are light at the start of the phase. However, by the fourth week, you should be "pumped" and hurting on the final sets. That doesn't mean you won't feel an effect in the first week or so, because you will, especially if you're not used to fast-paced training. Again, that's the idea. Your condition will improve from week to week, and you'll be ready to peak in week four.

As you'll see, there's a rhythm to the workouts just as there was in the entry-level routine. The sets drop from 3 to 2 in the last workout of each week. That's because you are repeating the day 1 workout, and will bring some accumulated fatigue to the workout on day 5. The cutback will help to avoid overtraining. You'll be ready to up the poundages at the start of the next week.

You will also note that the percentage doesn't increase in the third week. You drop back to the weights used in the first week, but the reps increase; in addition, the number of sets vary. The variety makes the workouts more interesting. What's more, the backoff in week three prepares you to max-out in the final week.

Study the workout chart, and you won't have any trouble following the training plan.

Once again, remember that 65/12-3 means 3 sets of 12 reps with 65% of your 12-rep maximum. If you don't know what you can lift in some of these exercises, experiment for a few days before starting the phase; an educated guess on the starting poundages is fine. Do a general warm-up at the start of each workout, and warm up for each exercise as necessary (see the

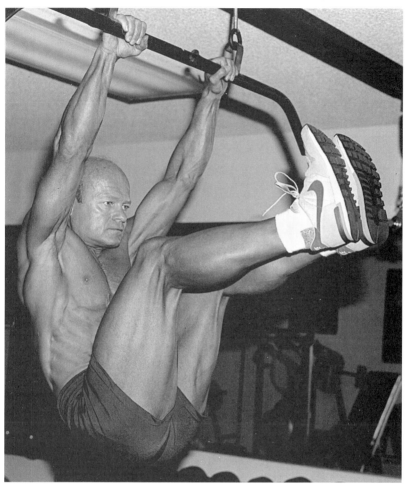

The Hanging Hip Curl, shown here, is included in one workout to complement the Abdominal Crunch in the other. The Crunch works the upper abs and the Hip Curl stresses the lower abs. Curl the hips up toward the rib cage and contact the lower abs as you lift your legs, hold briefly in the position shown here, and then lower slowly. Don't swing, because that takes stress off the abdominal muscles. *Photo by Guy Appelman.*

entry-level routine for details). Finally, remember that the rest period between sets is very important in volume training; rest 1-2 minutes between sets in this phase (see text).

Volume Phase

THE VOLUME PHASE

Exercise	Week One			Week Two			Week Three			Week Four		
Day	1	3	5	1	3	5	1	3	5	1	3	5
Barbell Squat	65/12-2		65/12-2	75/12-3		75/12-2	65/15-2		65/10-3	85/12-3		80/15-2
Bent-Knee Deadlift		65/12-3			75/12-3			65/12-2			85/12-3	
Standing Calf Raise	same		same	same		same	same		same	same		same
Seated Calf Raise		same			same			same			same	
One-Arm DB Row	same		same	same		same	same		same	same		same
Lat Pulldown (front)		same			same			same			same	
Barbell Bench Press	same		same	same		same	same		same	same		same
Incline DB Press		same			same			same			same	
Seat DB Press	same		same	same		same	same		same	same		same
Dumbbell Upright Row		same			same			same			same	
Barbell Curl	same		same	same		same	same		same	same		same
Narrow-grip Bench Press		same			same			same			same	
Abdominal Crunch	15-2		15-1	12-2		14-1	15-2		15-1	15-1		16-1
Hanging Hip Curl		10-2			18-2			10-2			22-1	

114

The Mixed Phase

The mixed phase is the second phase of the mass and strength routine. It's a mixture of volume training and strength training. Again it lasts 4 weeks. Half of the workouts are fast-paced volume, as in the last phase, and the other half are slow-paced, strength training.

The purpose of volume training is to deplete the muscles' energy stores, while the aim of strength training is to exhaust the contractile fibers. The main difference between the two types of training is the total number of reps and the amount of recovery allowed between sets.

Volume training demands that you do more total reps to get a "pump" and challenge the endurance components of the muscle. In strength training, you avoid the pump and burn, because they shut the muscles down before the contractile fibers are fully taxed. That's not what you want. Your objective in strength training is to directly fatigue the contractile fibers; you want to tire the muscle fibers so much that they can no longer lift the weight. To accomplish that requires that you keep the reps relatively low—to minimize the build-up of lactic acid—and rest long enough to allow complete recovery to occur between sets. In strength training, Dr. Bompa says, "Your last set should be as good as your first set."

In this phase, you only train twice a week. There are two whole-body workouts each week, one volume and one strength. The strength workout is always done first in the week, on day 1, and the volume workout is done on day 5.

In this phase, you only train twice a week. There are two whole-body workouts each week, one volume and one strength. The strength workout is always done first in the week, on day 1, and the volume workout is done on day 5. To the extent allowed by a seven-day week, that fits the recommended training frequencies, or work/rest ratios, mentioned earlier: three or four days rest after high-intensity, strength training and 48 hours after volume training. It also squares with my experience.

As I'll explain more fully in connection with my current routine, I've found through trial and error that I need about four days to recover from high-intensity weight workouts, and two or three days to recover from high-intensity aerobic sessions, which have much the same impact on the muscles as volume weight training.

Please note that there are two complementary workouts each week, one strength and one volume, and that each exercise is done in both styles an equal number of times. The strength workout is always done on day 1, however, because it takes longer to recover from strength workouts. That makes it necessary to repeat the same exercises in back-to-back workouts. The pattern is clear when you look at the chart.

Let's talk about poundages, or load pattern. You might be inclined to use the same weights here as in phase one when, for example, the chart calls for 80% of your 15 rep maximum in both phases. Remember, however, that this is "progressive" resistance training. As a result of your phase 1 training, you'll be stronger in this phase. Only you can judge how much stronger, but you should be able to handle more weight for 15 reps in this phase. If you did 200 pounds for two sets of 15 reps in the volume phase, perhaps you'll be ready to do 210 or even 220 here. The amount of improvement probably depends on how long you've been training. All I can do is urge you to train progressively. Try to lift more weight as you move from phase to phase and cycle to cycle. Progress is what makes weight training rewarding. That's the challenge.

While we are discussing poundages, I should mention that the load percentages are not written in stone. The workouts at the end of each phase should be hard, but not impossible. Feel free to adjust the percentages as necessary to fit your strength curve; some people are good at doing high reps and others, usually those with a high proportion of fast-twitch muscle fibers, excel at doing low reps. What's important is the change in load from week to week, the rhythm. Stick with the pattern, the recommended ups and downs in load from week to week. The systematic change of intensity that occurs in each phase is the key; that's what makes periodization work.

I don't time my rest intervals in strength workouts. I wait until I'm ready to exert maximum effort in the next set, and then I go for it.

One final point, and then you'll be ready to tackle the Mixed workouts. As you know, I suggest 60- to 120-second rest periods between sets in volume workouts. How long should the rest intervals be in strength training mode? Bompa suggests 3 to 5 minutes. That's probably about right, but I don't time my rest intervals in strength workouts. I wait until I'm ready to exert maximum effort in the next set, and then I go for it.

As mentioned before, you'll need more rest between sets on big-muscle exercises, such as Squats, than you will on Curls. Take the time you need, but don't cool off or let your mind wander. Keep moving. Concentrate. Stay focused. Enjoy the challenge of strength training.

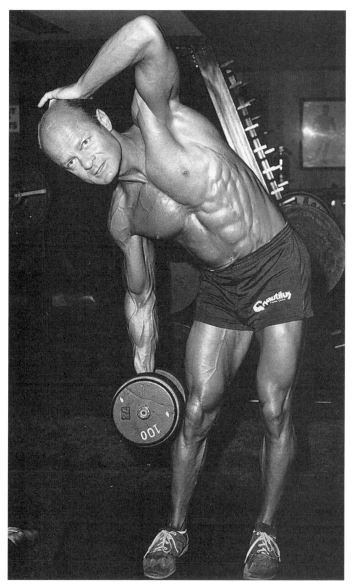

The Dumbbell Side Bend, shown here, is included in the mixed phase. Don't worry about overdeveloping your sides, or obliques. I've done this exercise for years, with only positive results. *Photo by Bill Reynolds.*

By the way, be sure to walk or do some other low-intensity aerobic activity on off days. It's okay to up the intensity of your aerobics a little on day 3, if you like. Just don't wear yourself out. Don't undercut your progress by doing too much. Allow yourself to recover fully between weight workouts.

THE MIXED PHASE

Exercise	Week One 1 (Stg)	Week One 5 (Vol)	Week Two 1 (Stg)	Week Two 5 (Vol)	Week Three 1 (Stg)	Week Three 5 (Vol)	Week Four 1 (Stg)	Week Four 5 (Vol)
Day	1 (Stg)	5 (Vol)	1 (Stg)	5 (Vol)	1 (Stg)	5 (Vol)	1 (Stg)	5 (Vol)
Barbell Squat	75/8-2			75/12-3	75/6-3			80/15-2
Bent-Knee Deadlift		65/12-3	85/8-2			65/15-2	95/8-2	
Standing Calf Raise	same		same		same		same	
Seated Calf Raise		same		same		same		same
Seated Cable Row	same		same		same		same	
Behind Neck Lat Pulldown		same		same		same		same
Bench Press	same		same		same		same	
Incline DB Press		same		same		same		same
Seated DB Press	same		same		same		same	
Upright Row		same		same		same		same
Dumbbell Curl	same		same		same		same	
Narrow-Grip Bench Press		same		same		same		same
Dumbbell Side Bend	15-1		15-1		15-1		18-1	
Hanging Hip Curl		12-2		12-2		12-2		18-1

Do general warm-up at the start of each workout, and warm up for each exercise as necessary (see entry-level routine for details). Rest 1-2 minutes between sets in volume sessions, and 3-5 minutes in strength sessions (see text). On DB Side Bend, use enough weight to make the last few reps difficult.

The Strength Phase

This is the third and final phase of the second routine. Obviously, the purpose of this phase is to build strength. But that's not all—the strength phase is also designed to build quality muscle. As you'll recall from the last chapter, Bompa and Poliquin agree that low-volume, high-intensity training is the best way to make the contractile fibers grow. In fact, Bompa says, "Maximum strength training... is the only way to improve chronic hypertrophy." In other words, strength training builds muscle that lasts.

According to Bompa, most bodybuilders use only volume training to build muscle mass. "What is very neglected," Bompa says, "is the type of training that stimulates the recruitment of [fast-twitch] muscle fibers to build high-density, tight muscle tone."

Building on the foundation of the other phases, this phase completes the picture. By stimulating the maximum possible number of muscle fibers, strength training adds good quality, striated muscle.

As in the last phase, there are two complementary whole-body workouts done only 2 days a week, again for four weeks. The difference is that all workouts are done in strength training mode. The rest periods between sets are 3-5 minutes, or as long as necessary to prepare for another maximum effort.

As in the last phase, there are two complementary whole-body workouts done only 2 days a week, again for four weeks. The difference is that all workouts are done in strength training mode. The rest periods between sets are 3-5 minutes, or as long as necessary to prepare for another maximum effort. The load percentages are higher and the reps are lower, because only heavy weights provide maximum stimulation to the fast-twitch fibers.

You'll note that there's a major difference in the frequency of these workouts and those recommended by Bompa and other proponents of periodization. The maximum strength training programs in Bompa's *Serious Strength Training* call for exercises to be repeated three or 4 times a week. I believe that's too much for most people.

Exercises here are done only once a week, and there are 3 or 4 days rest after each workout. That works for me, and I believe most bodybuilders will get better results with this lower training frequency. (See the discussion of the wound healing theory of recovery in the last chapter.)

Actually, I wish there were eight days in a week, so there could be four full days of rest after each strength workout. But we are stuck with a 7-day week. To compensate, we back off to 80% intensity in week 3. This gives the body a chance to recuperate and adapt in preparation for 3 sets of 4 reps at 95% in the final week.

As in the last phase, I suggest that you walk on off days to burn calories and speed recovery. Again, it's okay to increase the intensity of your aerobics on day 3, but don't wear yourself out.

A final tip before you begin. Concentrate. Don't hold back. Use your mind. Think "speed" even though the actual speed of movement will be slow because of the heavy weights used. Send a powerful message to every possible muscle fiber to contract for all it's worth.

That's what strength training is all about: conditioning the central nervous system to marshall the maximum possible number of motor units (nerve and muscle) to lift the weight. That's how you build strength—and muscle.

Not only that, but the improved ability to synchronize and recruit muscle fibers built in this final phase carries over and makes the volume phase in the next training cycle more productive. It's another virtuous circle; the volume and mixed phases prepare you to lift more in the strength phase as well. Ideally, the three phases working together create an almost never ending cycle of improvement.

That doesn't mean you should throw caution to the wind in the strength phase, however. Be careful. The weights will be heavy. You'll need a good warm-up for each exercise. Hold your position and control the weight at all times. Think "speed" but also think "safety."

Train progressively. Your goal should always be to start— and finish—each phase with more weight than the time before. Challenge yourself.

When you complete this phase, you'll be ready for a week or two of active rest. When your enthusiasm returns, there are at least two options. One is to repeat this phase with slightly heavier weights; that's a good idea because the strength phase is the most productive of the three phases. Don't do more than two strength phases, however, because this type of training is very taxing on the neuromuscular system.

The other option, probably the best one for most people, is to start the training cycle again, with the volume phase.

Remember, you're stronger now. Train progressively. Your goal should always be to start—and finish—each phase with more weight than the time before. Challenge yourself.

THE STRENGTH PHASE

Exercise	Week One		Week Two		Week Three		Week Four	
	Day 1	Day 5	Day 1	Day 5	Day 1	Day 5	Day 1	Day 5
Bent-Knee Deadlift	85/8-2		90/6-2		80/6-2		95/4-3	
Barbell Squat		85/8-2		90/6-2		80/6-2		95/4-3
Seated Calf Raise	same		same		same		same	
Standing Calf Raise		same		same		same		same
Lat Pulldown (front)	same		same		same		same	
Bent-Over Dumbbell Row		same		same		same		same
Incline Barbell Press	same		same		same		same	
Bench Press		same		same		same		same
Dumbbell Upright Row	same		same		same		same	
Seated DB Press		same		same		same		same
Narrow-Grip Bench Press	same		same		same		same	
Barbell Curl		same		same		same		same
Abdominal Crunch	30-1		35-1		30-1		40-1	
Hanging Hip Curl		15-1		20-1		15-1		25-1

Do general warm-up at start of each workout, and warm up for each exercise as necessary (see entry-level routine for details). Rest 3-5 minutes between sets, or as long as necessary to prepare for another maximum effort.

My Personal Weights/Aerobics Routine

This routine calls for weights on day 1 and aerobics on day 5. That's it.

It's the routine that gave me a physique as good—or better—at 60 than at 40. After seeing the outlines of the routine on our web site and in *IronMan* magazine, some have expressed the belief that this is a maintenance routine. That's not the case. As I said in chapter one, I don't believe in maintenance routines. *Challenge Yourself* is the name of this book. That's my overarching philosophy. I always train to get better. This routine is no exception.

Before I begin, be forewarned that my explanation why this routine works is a little long. I want to do my best to satisfy those who have serious doubts about training so infrequently and about the potency of doing only one work set. Those who are more interested in "how" than "why," may want to skip over this section and the next section, and perhaps come back later for the explanation.

Almost three decades after the publication of his landmark *Nautilus Training Principles*, Arthur Jones is reputed to have said that, given everything he now knows, if he were to do it again he would recommend training once per week on a whole-body routine. (He originally recommended training the whole body three times a week.) Whether or not Arthur actually said that, it expresses my belief about this routine. If I had it to do over again, I would start training with weights only once a week much earlier than I did. I'm convinced that my physique would've been better—at 30, 40, 50 and 60—if I had trained less frequently. For an advanced bodybuilder, I firmly believe that less truly is more.

Arthur Jones may initially have been a little overeager in prescribing training frequency, but I believe he was correct on the general principle. In *Bulletin No. 2*, published in 1971, Jones wrote: "Exactly contrary to the generally-practiced rule, advanced trainees should actually train less than they did earlier—but much harder."

For beginners, any exercise is an overload and promotes growth. As training progresses, however, it takes more and more intensity to promote growth. Furthermore, as Arthur counseled, "The amount of exercise must be decreased as the intensity of exercise is increased."

The maxim "You can train long or you can train hard, but you can't do both" applies with more force as one moves from beginner to intermediate to advanced status. The harder you train, the greater the impact on the system. An advanced trainer, therefore, needs more rest to allow the body to recover and rebuild itself bigger and stronger. With experience, training sessions must become shorter, harder—and less frequent.

David Staplin's wound healing theory of recovery, discussed in the last chapter, helps to explain the physiological details. As you'll recall, Staplin believes the wound healing process, especially the inflammatory response, provides a good model for studying and understanding muscle recovery. According to Staplin, high-intensity training damages the muscle cells. The degree of damage depends on the intensity of the exercise. "The higher the intensity, the greater the damage," says Staplin. What's more, Dave says, "It is the process of healing this damage which then makes the muscle cell large and stronger."

> **In the six-step healing process, the bottom line is that complete recovery can take five days or longer.**

I won't repeat the six-step healing process, but the bottom line is that complete recovery can take five days or longer. If the damage is severe enough, Staplin says healing can take up to six weeks! No weight workout is likely to cause that degree of trauma, of course, but it illustrates the importance of rest.

Staplin's application of wound healing theory to recovery finds support in the latest thinking of exercise physiologists on muscle soreness. Soreness occurs when a muscle is subjected to greater than normal stress, when it is overloaded. Since overload is a prerequisite for growth, I judge the effectiveness of my workouts based on soreness. Within limits, I welcome soreness, because it indicates that the complaining muscles are adapting, getting stronger and bigger in response to overload.

Consistent with my thinking and Staplin's theory, Professors Jack H. Wilmore and David A. Costill, in their textbook *Physiology of Sport and Exercise* (Human Kinetics, 1994), say, "We are now confident that muscle soreness results from injury or damage to the muscle itself." Significantly, they add, "Some evidence suggests that this process is an important step in muscle hypertrophy."

To further test that view, I contacted Dr. Lucille Smith, a professor at Appalachian State University and an internationally recognized expert on exercise-induced muscle damage. I asked Professor Smith whether it is advisable to train again before soreness subsides. This is important, of course, because Staplin maintains that training again before the healing process is complete short-circuits recovery and nips supercompensation in the bud.

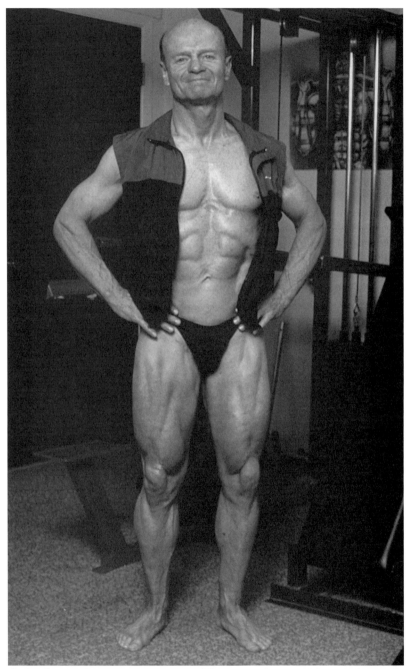

If I had it to do over again, I would start training with weights only once a week earlier than I did. I'm convinced that my physique would've been better—at 30, 40, 50 and 60—if I had trained less frequently. *Photo by Pat Berrett.*

That's why I do only one weight workout a week. To insure that the growth process has run its course, I don't train again until a few days after the soreness is gone.

Understandably, Dr. Smith didn't commit herself completely, because the precise causes of muscle damage and the process of repair are not fully understood. Still, her response was consistent with Dave Staplin's theory of recovery—and my rationale for training with weights only once a week.

> It appears that soreness is the body's way of discouraging us from doing anything that would interfere with the healing and growth process.

Dr. Smith said, "I'm not sure that soreness totally reflects the underlying tissue condition, [but] I think it occurs to reduce activity during a critical time of healing."

Clearly, that supports the wisdom of not training again until the soreness is gone, especially in view of the fact that Wilmore and Costill suggest that the "healing" is an important step in muscle growth. It appears that soreness is the body's way of discouraging us from doing anything that would interfere with the healing and growth process.

Smith seems to agree, because she added: "The thing that impresses me is that you are getting stronger. This has to be a positive adaptation." (I'm usually a little stronger when I repeat the same workout, and I'm almost never weaker.)

She expressed surprise, however, that I get sore every time I train, "since the research literature suggests that once you have experienced soreness, you are 'protected' for about 6 weeks for the same intensity. This is called the repeated bout effect." Happily, she concurred with my explanation: "As you suggested, it might be that you are able to workout at a much greater intensity."

Again, I believe that soreness indicates that my workouts are successful, that I am overloading my muscles.

Reinforcing Lucille Smith's surmise—and my interpretation— Professors McArdle, Katch and Katch, in the fourth edition of their textbook *Exercise Physiology* (Williams & Wilkins, 1996), say the repeated bout effect "does not provide complete protection from subsequent soreness with more intense exercise."

My training schedule is designed to keep my soreness and my workouts in proper balance. I usually do my weight workout at about 11:00 in the morning on Sunday. I start to feel stiff and inflamed by evening.

Remember that Staplin says muscle cell damage, the first step in the process, causes an inflammatory response, which in turn causes further damage and soreness. I can vouch for that, because I feel more inflamed and stiff the next day, on Monday.

Specific muscle soreness usually peaks on Tuesday, the second day after the workout. (That's why exercise-induced soreness is generally called delayed-onset muscle soreness.) I'm almost always sore in the traps, lower back, gluts, quads, hamstrings, calves, upper back, chest, shoulders and triceps, every place but my biceps, which rarely get sore. (My biceps just don't seem to be wired to allow maximum stimulation.)

The soreness usually starts to subside by Wednesday. While the soreness is gone by Thursday, I still don't feel recovered enough for another weight session. But I am ready for my high-intensity aerobic workout on day 5.

I got the idea that I can do hard aerobics even though I'm not ready for another weight session from Vladimir M. Zatsiorsky, Ph.D., the famed Soviet sports scientist who is now a professor at Penn State. In his book *Science and Practice of Strength Training* (Human Kinetics, 1995), Zatsiorsky says that "fatigue effects from different types of muscular work are specific." According to Zatsiorsky, that means you might not be recovered enough to do a heavy strength workout, but you may very well be sufficiently recovered for a hard aerobics session. I've found that to be true.

> **I feel depleted after my aerobics session, but I don't get sore, suggesting that high-intensity aerobics does not cause muscle damage.**

I recover faster from high-intensity aerobics than from weights. I feel depleted after my aerobics session, but I don't get sore, suggesting that high-intensity aerobics does not cause muscle damage. When Sunday rolls around, three days after my aerobics session and a full week following my weight session, I'm usually ready to launch into another heavy resistance session. On occasion, however, I've rested another week, when I didn't feel recovered, and always come back stronger.

That's the reasoning behind my current once-a-week training schedule. Before we get to the actual workouts, however, I promised to tell you about new research on the efficacy of doing only one hard set of each exercise (after warmup). I've long favored this approach, and—with one exception I'll explain shortly—I use it in this routine.

One Set or Many Sets?

As explained earlier, there's strong evidence that both one-set and multi-sets work—but for different reasons. Multiple sets of each exercise done at a fast pace—the form of training described in the last routine—build muscular endurance and size by increasing energy stores. Whereas, high-intensity, single-set training builds strength and muscular hypertrophy by enlarging the contractile proteins, primarily the powerful fast-twitch fibers.

Nevertheless, nothing stirs up more controversy than the sets issue, not only among athletes but also in the academic world.

"Just one set of each strength exercise, correctly done twice a week, is generally enough to increase strength significantly," commented the editors of *Physician and Sportsmedicine* (February,1997).

"Monumental misinformation," Howard G. Knuttgen, Ph.D. of University Park, Pennsylvania, fired back. According to Dr. Knuttgen, the correct prescription for active adults is "2 or 3 sets repetition maximum per session for each muscle group" done "3 to 4 sessions per week." (*PSM*, May 1997) And that wasn't the end of it.

Dr. Ralph N. Carpinelli, who teaches the neuromuscular aspects of strength training at Adelphi University, Long Island, N. Y., took up Dr. Knuttgen's challenge in Richard Winett's *Master Trainer* (Feb 1998). "There is no scientific evidence, nor is there any physiological basis, that would support the superiority of multiple sets," wrote Dr. Carpinelli. "Theoretically," he continued, "as people become stronger and wish to attain maximal increases in strength and hypertrophy, which is not accomplished without optimal recuperation, they may require *lower* volume and frequency."

Carpinelli, who did an extensive review of the scientific literature on one set versus many, believes "the quantity of exercise is not as important as the quality of exercise." (*Master Trainer*, December 1997).

I agree with Dr. Carpinelli, but I see value in both methods. It really boils down to specificity, the guiding principle of all athletic training. According to this time honored principle, the body's response to stress is specific adaptation to imposed demand (SAID).

As I've said several times, you can train hard or you can train long, but you can't do both. In other words, volume and intensity are mutually exclusive. It is difficult, perhaps impossible, to maintain quality—or intensity—and do many sets. In *Lean For Life*, I explained how this works in actual practice. When you plan to do multiple work sets, consciously or subconsciously, you pace yourself; you hold back on the early sets,

The outcome is predictable, based on the SAID principle. Multiple sets build endurance and single sets build strength.

saving energy for the sets to follow. Like a long-distance runner, you husband your strength.

On the other hand, do only one set and you can focus totally on that set without thinking about the sets to come. You are free to make an all-out effort, you don't have to hold anything in reserve. As in the 100-yard dash, you give it all you've got from start to finish. The result is a more intense set, which forces more muscle fibers into action.

The outcome is predictable, based on the SAID principle. Multiple sets build endurance and single sets build strength.

By imposing a specific demand on the contractile fibers, namely to lift a heavy weight as many times as possible, one-set training recruits the maximum number of fibers, causing them to adapt by becoming bigger and stronger.

By the same token, subjecting the muscles to the repeated demands of multiple sets forces them to adapt by building additional energy stores. The result is bigger and more enduring muscles, capable of doing set after set.

As Arthur Drechsler observes in *The Weightlifting Encyclopedia* (A Is A, 1998), whether one set or multiple sets are best depends on what you're trying to accomplish. For instance, if you are training for an event that requires repeated bouts of effort, multiple sets are probably indicated.

The number of reps in a set also has a bearing on the appropriate number of sets. Drechsler says, "There is now scientific evidence that more muscle fibers are activated on a maximum set of [five, ten or 20] reps than on a maximum single. From this it follows that a maximum set of high reps is more likely to stimulate a maximum training effect than a maximum single."

> A review of literature by Carpinelli and Otto found that 33 out of 35 strength-training studies showed no significant difference in strength or size gains as a result of doing one set or multiple sets

Competitive weightlifters, Artie's primary focus, who perform relatively low reps in training, will typically need to do multiple sets.

For much the same reason, the optional Power Snatches and Power Cleans included in this routine are performed for several sets. These quick lifts are typically done in sets of five reps or less, because the speed and coordination required tend to break down when more reps are employed.

Bodybuilders, who are mainly concerned with muscle size, can profitably employ one set, many sets, or a combination. (If you overtrain, of course, no approach will work very well.)

128

These points may help to explain why research on the optimum number of sets has been inconclusive. A review of literature by Carpinelli and Otto found that 33 out of 35 strength-training studies showed no significant difference in strength or size gains as a result of doing one set or multiple sets (*Sports Medicine*, 25(7): 1998). The two main criticisms of these studies, according to Dr. Carpinelli, are that they were too short, and that the participants were often untrained. The suggestion is that seasoned trainers might benefit from doing more sets.

Those criticisms, which Dr. Carpinelli termed "valid" in the October 1998 *Master Trainer*, are addressed in a series of five studies by Michael Pollock, M.D., and his colleagues at the University of Florida, and another study by Dr. K.L. Ostrowski's research group.

Four of the Pollock-group studies address the duration issue; they extend for six months compared to only six to 12 weeks in the earlier studies. The last Pollock study and the study by Ostrowski and colleagues tackle the experience issue.

The new evidence is interesting and, I believe, lends support to the thesis that one set training builds strength and multisets build endurance. What's more, it challenges the belief that, for experienced trainers, more is better.

Two of the Pollock studies (*Medicine and Science in Sports and Exercise*, Supplement 30(5); 116 & 165, 1998) examine strength and size increases as a result of one set or three sets of 8–12 repetitions to muscular failure three days a week. Strength was assessed for both one rep max and reps at 75 percent of pretraining max, in the Bench Press, Row, Arm Curl, Leg Extension and Leg Curl. Muscle thickness increases were measured by ultrasound in eight locations covering the upper and lower body.

The researchers found almost identical increases in upper and lower body thickness for both the one-set (13.6%) and three-set (13.12%) groups. Increases in one-rep maximum were also essentially the same for all five exercises, but the principle of specificity asserted itself on one exercise when it came to maximum reps, or endurance. Both groups showed significant across-the-board increases in endurance, but the three-set group showed significantly greater improvement in the Bench Press. At 25 weeks, the one-set group averaged 22 reps compared to 27 for those doing three sets, a difference of 23 percent.

The third 6-month study by the Pollock group (*Medicine and Science in Sports and Exercise*, Supplement 30(5): S163, 1998) focused on increases in knee-extensions strength in three different modes: one-rep max, isometric peak torque and training weight. Again, there was no significant difference between the one-set and three-set groups. One-rep max increased 33.3% and 31.6% for 1 set and 3 sets, respectively; isometric increases were 35.4% versus 32.1%; and training weight increases were 25.6% compared to 14.7%.

Even though the researchers apparently didn't find it significant, note that the one-set group gained slightly more strength

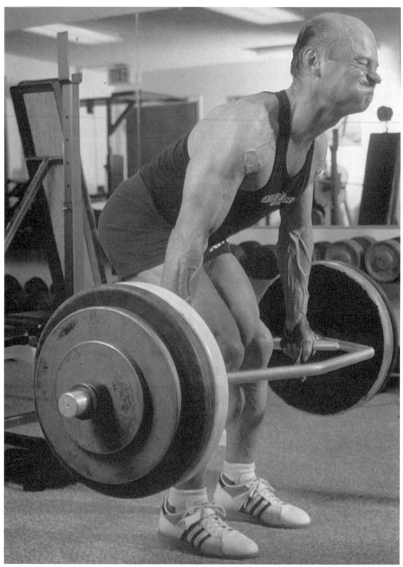

When you do only one set there's nothing to keep you from going all-out, but when you plan to do three sets it's natural to hold back and pace yourself. *Photo by Pat Berrett.*

in the first two modes and substantially more in training weight (25.6% versus 14.7%). It seems that specificity is at work again. When you do only one set there's nothing to keep you from going all-out, but when you plan to do three sets it's natural to hold back and pace yourself. That's probably why the one-set group gained more strength; they triggered more muscle fibers than the 3-set group, where pacing was probably a factor.

The fourth study by the Pollock group (*Medicine and Science in Sports and Exercise*, Supplement 30(5): S274, 1998) also six months long, showed significant increases in circulating insulin-like growth factors (IGFs) in both one-set (34%) and three-set (30%) groups. (Dr. Carpinelli, who teaches the neuromuscular aspects of strength training, says "IGFs are multifunctional protein hormones, whose production in the liver and other tissues is stimulated by growth hormones." Carpinelli says IGFs are important, because "they stimulate glucose and amino acid uptake, protein and DNA synthesis, and growth of bones, cartilage, and soft tissue.")

> Some have suggested that experienced trainers might benefit from higher volume. According to this study, those people should think anew.

The researchers concluded: "The elevation of IGFs is no greater with high- than low-volume resistance training."

The final study by the Pollock group (*Medicine and Science in Sports and Exercise*, Supplement 30(5): S115, 1998) addresses the training experience issue. As you'll recall, some have suggested that experienced trainers might benefit from higher volume. In other words, after you've been training for a while, you need greater volume to progress; more is better. According to this study, those people should think anew.

The researchers recruited 40 adults who had been training for a minimum of one year; average training time was six years. The participants were randomly assigned to either a one-set or three-set group; both groups did 8-12 reps to failure three days per week for 13 weeks.

Both groups significantly increased their one-rep maximum strength and their endurance. There was no significant difference in the gains made by the two groups in the Leg Extension, Leg Curl, Bench Press, Overhead Press and Arm Curl. The researchers concluded: "These data indicate that 1 set of [resistance training] is equally as beneficial as 3 sets in experienced resistance trained adults."

K.L. Ostrowski and colleagues tested "the effect of weight training volume on hormonal output and muscular size and function" in experienced trainers (*Journal of Strength and Conditioning Research* 11(3): 148-154, 1997). Thirty-five males, with one to four years weight-training experience, were assigned to one of three training groups: one set, two sets, or four sets. All participants did what I would call a periodized program; the rep range was changed every few weeks. They did six free-weight exercises four times a week for ten weeks using 12 rep maximum (week 1–4), 7 reps (week 5–7) and 9 reps (week 8–10). All sets were performed to muscular fatigue with three minutes rest between sets. The only difference between the three programs was the number of sets.

As in the Pollock group studies, no significant differences were found. The authors concluded: "...A low volume program...[one set of each exercise]...results in increases in muscle size and function similar to programs with two to four times as much volume."

Significantly, regarding hormone output, they concluded: "High volume [four sets of each exercise] may result in a shift in the testosterone/cortisol (anabolic/catabolic) ratio in some individuals, suggesting the possibility of overtraining." In other words, high-volume training may lead to overtraining, especially in the case of experienced lifters.

After considering this new evidence, Dr. Carpinelli issued his verdict: "The lack of scientific evidence that multiple sets... produce a greater increase in strength or size, in itself, provides a rationale for following a single set training protocol."

I warned you that the explanation would be long. I hope I've allayed the doubts I know many have about infrequent, one-set training. It has worked very well for me. Now, it's finally time to cut to the chase. Here's the routine I followed to peak at 60.

The Weight Workouts

The entire routine, weights and aerobics, is an advanced version of the A-B, whole-body, balanced routine in *Lean For Life*. We've already discussed many of the elements in the first two routines. One difference here, of course, is the inclusion of high-intensity aerobics, which we'll discuss in the next section. If you need further clarification after reading my explanation, there's an expanded discussion of the basic elements of this routine in *Lean For Life*.

You already know this routine calls for only one work set (after warm up), and that there is only one weight session each week. Workout A is done one week and workout B the next. Other than that, the main difference between this routine and the routine in *Lean For Life* is the intensity of the workouts.

132

You might say this is a hybrid of the HIT system, which calls for training to failure every workout, and periodization, where training is done in phases, which gradually build to maximum poundages over a period of weeks.

Working out only once a week makes it possible to maintain a very high level of intensity, but it's important to note that I don't strive for PRs every workout. That would be a mistake. Training to failure creates the encore problem discussed in my other books; attempting to top yourself every time you go to the gym saps enthusiasm and inevitably leads to sticking points. I believe constantly training to failure is both physiologically and psychologically unsound. It's a prescription for failure.

> **To make progress, an advanced trainer needs both high-intensity and the planned change of periodization. This routine provides both.**

To make progress, an advanced trainer needs both high-intensity and the planned change of periodization. This routine provides both.

Intensity remains high all the time, but increases come only at the end of each phase. Like the routines in *Ripped 3* and *Lean For Life*, there are three phases: the endurance phase (20 reps per set), the strength and endurance phase (12-reps), and the strength phase (8 reps). The poundages, of course, increase as the reps decrease.

The plan is to achieve a modest new high in each exercise for 20 reps, then for 12 reps and finally 8 reps. After a short break, you're ready to begin again at 20 reps and so on. The net result is you consolidate your gains over the course of each three phase cycle, which sets the stage for further improvement. Slowly but surely, you improve from cycle to cycle.

This is a more realistic plan than simply sticking to one rep range and attempting to make gains every workout, especially for someone who's been training for years.

Experienced trainers know you can't lift more every time out, no matter how long you rest between workouts. It just won't happen, at least not for long. If it was possible to make gains every workout, many of us would be lifting skyscrapers by now.

On the other hand, coaxing gains as called for in this routine, attempting to increase a little every cycle, is realistic. You won't always achieve your goal, and you may have to repeat a cycle or even back off some from time to time. You won't be lifting any tall buildings, but your workouts will be satisfying. You'll still be progressing long after others have retired.

Here's how it works. Start each phase with your recent best.

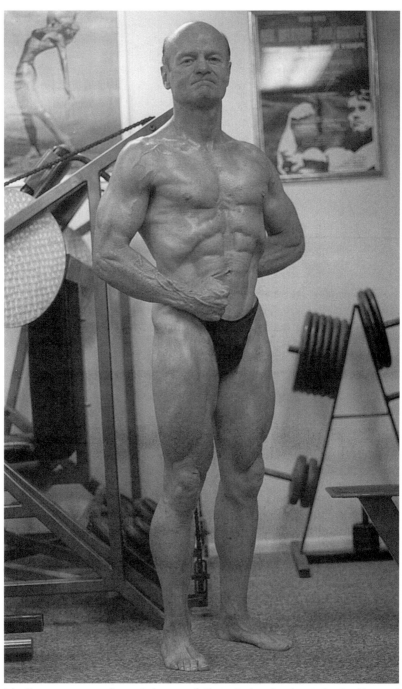

I believe constantly training to failure is both physiologically and pychologically unsound. It's a prescription for failure. *Photo by Pat Berrett.*

(Be realistic. Allow a little margin for error. Don't bite off more than you can chew.) If you're currently capable of doing 20 reps with 200 pounds in the Squat (workout A) and 225 in the Deadlift (workout B), those are the weights to use in weeks 1 and 2, respectively, of the endurance phase. In weeks 3 and 4, increase the weights about 2 percent, which would work out to 205 in the Squat and 230 in the Deadlift.

What about weeks 5 and 6? Do you go for more 20-rep records? No, that wouldn't be prudent. Instead, move on to the next phase, the 12-rep strength-and-endurance phase.

Let's assume your recent best efforts for 12 reps in the Squat and Deadlift, respectively, are 225 and 250. (Again, be realistic. Don't overreach.) Use those weights in weeks 5 and 6; and then, in weeks 7 and 8, move up again, perhaps to 230 in the Squat and 255 in the Deadlift.

Again, don't push your luck by trying to do more weight for 12 reps. If you've been lifting for some time, that wouldn't be wise. Move on to the strength phase, where the reps per set are eight.

By now you know how it works. In weeks 9 and 10, repeat your recent—and conservative—best for eight reps in each exercise, and then, in the next two weeks, raise the weights slightly; go for modest new 8-rep highs.

The beauty of this periodization scheme is that each phase prepares you to move up in the next phase. The new highs made for eight reps lay the groundwork for you to move up again in the next cycle.

After a few extra days rest, you'll be ready for another 20-rep phase. Begin with the poundages you used at the end of the last endurance phase—and you're off again. See the pattern? Repeat your previous high in each lift—to give your body and your mind a chance to adjust to the new strength level—before you attempt to move up.

Now that you know how the routine works, all you need is the other exercises in the A and B workouts. Here they are:

Workout A	Workout B
Power Snatch (optional)	Power Clean (optional)
Squat	Deadlift
Standing Calf Raise	Seated Calf Raise
Bent-over Dumbbell Row	Lat Pulldown
Bench Press	Incline Dumbbell Press
Seated Dumbbell Press	Parallel Bar Dip
Barbell Curl	Triceps Extension Behind Neck
Ab Crunches	Hanging Hip Curl

That's it. The key is to do a limited number of "big" exercises.

Stick to exercises that work a lot of muscles at one time. That way you can train your whole body very hard in one workout of manageable length.

Two different workouts allow you to train each body part more completely, but it also serves another purpose. It gives the body more time to recover and build before the next load increase. For example, the Squat and Deadlift work essentially the same muscles, but the angle of stress is different. Doing these exercises in alternative weeks, gives the massive muscles of the hips, lower back, frontal thighs and hamstrings more time to adapt in preparation to lift heavier weights.

Subjecting the body to roughly the same stresses throughout the 12-week training cycle, by using different poundage and rep combinations, serves the same purpose. Dr. Bompa explains why this is necessary: "One workout provides insufficient stimulus to produce marked changes in the body. Such adaptations occur only after repeated exposure to the same training loads."

This routine, with its long rest periods between workouts and judicious application of stress, fills the bill.

The Quick Lifts

Before we move on to the aerobics workouts, I want to say a few words about the Power Snatch and Clean, the optional quick lifts. We discussed athletic-type lifts in the last chapter, noting the important role they play in modern-day sports and their positive effect on John Grimek's magnificent physique.

Arthur Jones wrote that exercise movements should be performed as rapidly as possible, "but not during the first three or four repetitions," which he considered the most dangerous. Arthur warned that all competitive lifters, who of necessity must exert maximum power on the first rep, "are almost certain to hurt themselves sooner or later."

For better or worse, there's only one way to do the Power Snatch and Power Clean: quickly. That, of course, is why they're called quick lifts. To perform these lifts properly, you have to move fast—on every rep. But it's a controlled application of power. Maximum force is exerted only at the proper time. The weight comes off the floor slowly, under complete control, and it's only when the bar reaches a position between the knees and the hips, the position of maximum leverage, that the lifter explodes.

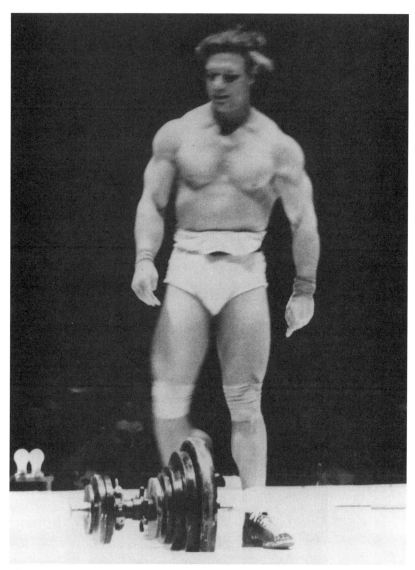

This rare, slightly out-of-focus photo of John Grimek in competition at the 1936 Olympic Games in Berlin, shows the ruggedly powerful physique he developed with the aid of the quick lifts. *Photo courtesy of the Todd-McLean Collection.*

Dr. Pat O'Shea, the author of *Quantum Strength*, says, "There is only minimal risk involved as long as you execute the...lifts utilizing good technique and lift within your age-related physical limits." Significantly, O'Shea adds: "As we age, athletic-type lifting contributes most to maintaining a high level of functional

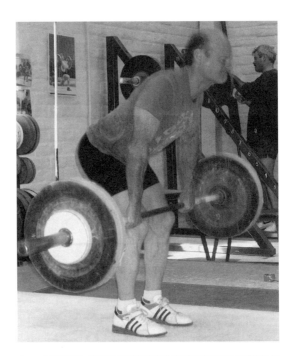

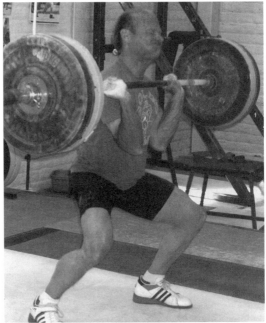

These photos show me doing the Power Clean. The weight comes off the floor slowly, under complete control, and it is only when the bar reaches a position above the knees that the lifter explodes upward and racks (catches) the bar on the shoulders. *Photo by Carl Miller.*

living through each decade of life." In other words, athletic-type lifts become more—not less—important with age.

That's why I do the quick lifts. (They're fun, too.) Athletic-type lifts, such as the Power Snatch and Power Clean—along with the Squat and Deadlift—are the first exercises in this routine, and an integral part of my training. They are the core of all my current workouts.

Nevertheless, there's no getting around the fact that there is some risk of injury involved in doing the quick lifts, especially if you are over 30 and have never done the Snatch and Clean before. That's why they are optional. The choice is yours.

It's beyond the scope of this book to explain all that's involved in safely learning the quick lifts. It requires patience, time and lots of practice.

If you are interested, I suggest that you read Dr. O'Shea's *Quantum Strength* and the relevant parts of *The Weightlifting Encyclopedia* by Arthur Drechsler; both books are available from Ripped Enterprises. Even though I taught myself how to do the quick lifts years ago by looking at still photos, it would be extremely helpful to see motion pictures of the lifts. You can rent or buy an excellent video presentation called "The Power Clean and Variations" from Bigger Faster Stronger, Inc.; call 1-800-628-9737.

As explained earlier, the quick lifts are typically done in sets of five reps or less. It's difficult to maintain proper form when you do more reps; it's like trying to run the 100-yard dash for a mile.

I do five reps in the endurance phase, three reps in the strength and endurance phase, and singles in the strength phase. I generally do only one set with the top weight—most competitive lifters probably do more sets, but I want to save my energy for the rest of the workout—but more sets than usual in working up to the target poundage. For example, after limbering up with a broom handle and the empty bar, I might do warm-up sets of 3, 2, 2, 1 and 1 with progressively heavier weights, before doing the target set. Like the other exercises in my routine, I only do enough to prepare my muscles, joints and my mind—mental preparation is critical for lifts which involve coordination of the whole body—for a maximum effort. As always, warm up, but don't wear yourself out.

Now, let's move on to the high-intensity aerobics portion of the routine.

The High-Intensity Aerobics Workouts

In the last chapter, I explained why the oft heard advice to "stay in the fat-burn zone" is misguided. Cutting-edge research shows that high intensity intervals are best for both fitness and fat loss. You don't stop burning fat when exercise intensity goes above the so called fat-burn zone, as many have been lead to believe; you burn the same amount of fat—and more calories. More importantly, the high-intensity approach conditions your body to burn fat more readily 24-hours a day.

As you know, this routine calls for one hard aerobics workout per week. That's it. The weight session is on day 1 and the aerobics session is on day 5. That allows four days of recovery after weights and three after aerobics. In accordance with the barbell strategy explained in the last chapter, I recommend comfortable walking on the off days, to burn fat and aid—not delay—recovery.

My aerobics workouts are modified versions of the Tabata and Tremblay interval protocols, which we discussed at length in the last chapter. As you'll remember, the Tabata intervals are very short (20 seconds work and 10 seconds rest), and the Tremblay intervals include longer work periods (60 to 90 seconds), separated by relatively long rest periods, allowing the heart rate to drop to about 120 beats per minute.

The two protocols, one with long intervals and the other with short, dovetail nicely with the weight workouts, which begin with 20-rep sets and progress to 12 reps and finally 8 reps, with progressively heavier weights. Here we pair the longer Tremblay intervals with the 20-rep phase and the shorter and more intense Tabata intervals with the 8-rep phase. We marry the two protocols and do mid-range intervals with the 12-rep strength-and-endurance phase.

Before we get to specific details, I want to repeat a warning issued by the Tremblay group—and echoed by Dr. Tabata in a personal communication with Richard Winett: *"High Intensity exercise cannot be prescribed for individuals at risk for health problems or for obese people who are not used to exercise."* If you have any doubts whatsoever about your health status, or if you have not been exercising regularly, DO NOT TRY THESE WORKOUTS WITHOUT CHECKING WITH YOUR DOCTOR.

The workouts here are similar to the aerobics workouts in *Lean For Life*, which utilize the Schwinn Air-Dyne stationary bicycle, the Concept II rowing machine and a treadmill with adjustable grade. Those machines are ideal for intervals, but any device that allows you to change the intensity quickly and easily will do fine. (You can, of course, do intervals outside; all you need are running shoes and a stop watch.) The Air-Dyne and the Concept II are especially good, because you make your own resistance by pedalling or rowing with more or less effort. The treadmill, however, doesn't allow you to change the intensity as easily and quickly. I solve that problem by setting the speed and grade beforehand—I warm up first, of course—and then stepping on the moving tread for the work intervals, and off for the rest periods. During rest periods, I straddle the moving tread and hold on to the bar at the front of the treadmill. (For those who need it, there are more tips on using the Air-Dyne, the Concept II and the treadmill in *Lean For Life*.)

I prefer to use a variety of aerobic equipment, because it spreads the stress to different areas of the body. As I explained in *Lean For Life*, if you want whole-body fitness, you have to train your whole body. While the heart and lungs benefit from

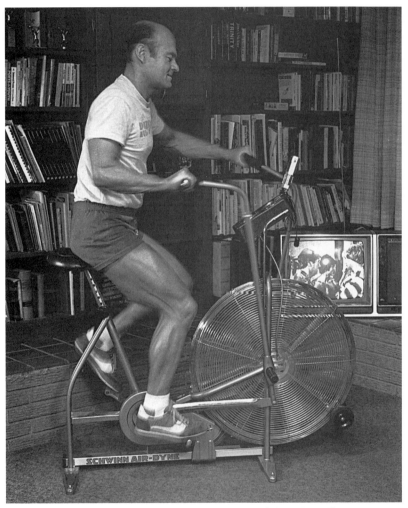

The Schwinn Air-Dyne incorporates a wonderful push-pull arm action, which spreads the fat-burning and conditioning benefits to the upper body as well as the lower. *Photo by Guy Appelman.*

any form of endurance exercise, that's not true of the muscles themselves. It's only the involved muscles that benefit.

I like the Air-Dyne and the Concept II because they work the upper body as well as the lower. (For those who don't know, the Air-Dyne incorporates a wonderful push-pull arm action.) Combining the Air-Dyne, the Concept II and the treadmill spreads the fat-burning and conditioning benefits of aerobic exercise all over the body. Spreading the stress in this manner also allows you to tolerate more aerobic exercise. (Again, for more details on the benefits of a varied, whole-body approach to aerobics, see *Lean For Life*.)

> I start all workouts with a 5-minute warm-up, followed by 5 minutes at a steady pace (fast enough to be hard at the end), and then I do another 5 minutes easy, before beginning the intervals. I always end with a 5-minute cooldown.

Here are the workouts. In sync with the weight sessions, the work intervals are long in the endurance phase (90 seconds), medium length in the strength and endurance phase (45 seconds) and short in the strength phase (20 seconds). The intervals, of course, become more intense as well. Just as a 20-rep set must be done with a lighter weight than an 8-rep set, a 90-second interval must be performed at a slower pace than a 20-second interval. Note, too, that there are four workouts using each piece of equipment. As I just explained, that helps to spread the stress over the whole body.

Endurance Phase

Week 1	Air-Dyne	4 x 90 seconds + 90s rest
Week 2	Treadmill	4 x 90 seconds + 90s rest
Week 3	Air-Dyne	5 x 90 seconds + 90s rest
Week 4	Treadmill	5 x 90 seconds + 90s rest

Strength and Endurance Phase

Week 5	Rower	6 x 45 seconds + 30s rest
Week 6	Treadmill	6 x 45 seconds + 30s rest
Week 7	Rower	7 x 45 seconds + 30s rest
Week 8	Treadmill	7 x 45 seconds + 30s rest

Strength Phase

Week 9	Air-Dyne	8 x 20 seconds + 10s rest
Week 10	Rower	8 x 20 seconds + 10s rest
Week 11	Air-Dyne	10 x 20 seconds + 10s rest
Week 12	Rower	10 x 20 seconds + 10s rest

As you'll remember, the Tabata and Tremblay study participants exercised 4 or 5 days a week. Because we do the protocols only once a week—to allow complete recovery from the weight sessions—I add a steady-state segment not shown above.

I start all workouts with a 5-minute warm-up, followed by 5 minutes at a steady pace (fast enough to be hard at the end), and then I do another 5 minutes easy, before beginning the intervals. I always end with a 5-minute cooldown. That makes the endurance phase sessions about 35 minutes in length and the strength phase workouts about 25 minutes; the strength and endurance sessions are in between, at a little under 30 minutes.

The actual pace of the workouts will vary from person to person. The Tabata group did the 20-second intervals at 170% of VO_2max, but VO_2max can only be measured in the laboratory. I simply experiment and find a pace that makes the last interval very hard to complete.

I also track my heart rate with a Polar chest-strap monitor. My heart rate is usually over 90 percent of my measured maximum, which is 190, at the end of the steady-state segment and again on the last interval. As my condition improves, of course, I increase the pace of the workouts. The best approach is to start conservatively and gradually up the intensity. (*Again, don't try this without first checking with your doctor.*)

The standard formula for estimating maximum heart rate is your age subtracted from 220. That means my maximum should be 160 (220 minus 60). As indicated, my measured maximum is actually 190. Yours may vary from the norm as well. Some very well conditioned athletes have lower heart rates and others, like me, have a higher max. Experiment and you'll soon learn if your heart rate is higher or lower than expected. The main thing is to be sure that you're working hard at the end of the steady-state segment and on the last interval.

Believe it or not, I've come to enjoy these brief, but hard interval workouts. I like the challenge—and seeing my condition improve over time. Still, I don't believe I'd enjoy doing hard intervals more than once a week, especially when I'm also training hard with weights.

Coming to workouts well rested is great for your enthusiasm. If you try this routine, don't give in to the temptation to train more often. You'll progress faster—and stay motivated longer—if you remember that "less is more."

By the way, don't forget to walk on a regular basis. I walk for an hour or more on off days, in one long walk or 2 or 3 shorter walks. I also walk for at least 20 minutes on workout days. Comfortable walking is a very important part of my lifetime plan to stay lean. I suggest that you make walking (or something similar) part of your life as well.

Have fun!

An Ongoing Process

Continuing my decades-long trend toward less frequent training, I've just begun experimenting with a 9-day training cycle. I do this reluctantly, because of the convenience of training on the same days each week; but my body was telling me that a regular 7-day week was not allowing the rest necessary for continued progress. I simply did not feel completely recovered when it came time to train again; I still felt a residual soreness and a lingering sense of fatigue.

> **I have added an extra day of rest after both weight and aerobics sessions. I now rest 5 days (120 hours) after weights and 4 days (96 hours) after aerobics.**

As mentioned, I tried resting an extra week from time to time—with positive results—but, more often than not, I still didn't feel quite ready to train again on a 7-day cycle. The fact that I almost always came back stronger after an extra week of rest—on one particularly memorable occasion, I broke a stubborn sticking point in the Power Snatch—gave me the confidence to break out of the confines of the 7-day week.

Moving slowly, as always, I have added an extra day of rest after both weight and aerobics sessions. I now rest 5 days (120 hours) after weights and 4 days (96 hours) after aerobics. For instance, if I train with weights on Sunday, I now do aerobics on Friday (rather than Thursday); my next weight session now comes on the following Tuesday, rather than Sunday. On a 9-day schedule, of course, my training days change every week.

It seems to be working fine, but I haven't been on the new schedule long enough to make a definitive assessment. All I can say is, so far so good. The extra rest days feel good. I look forward to training sessions more than ever.

I've also added a C workout to my schedule, which means I now repeat workouts every 27 days, rather than every two weeks, as I did under the A-B routine described in the last few sections. The reason for the change was to allow more time to work on the Squat Snatch.

The Squat Snatch is truly acrobatics with a barbell. The bar is pulled slightly above hip level, and then, in a lightning fast move, caught overhead in the full squat position.

Frankly, relearning the movement, after a lapse of more than 20 years, has been more difficult than I anticipated. I've found that, unlike riding a bicycle, the Squat Snatch isn't a movement you never forget. I tried practicing my form after aerobics, but I was too tired and missed more reps than I made. I also tried practicing on the days before and after my aerobics session, but that didn't work either; it interfered with recovery.

My solution has been to build an entirely new workout around the Squat Snatch. That allows me to devote more time and energy to mastering the Snatch, which requires more sets and reps than exercises where form is not an issue. In addition to about 30 minutes of Squat Snatches, my new C workout includes Barbell Squats, Ab Crunches, Chin-ups and Push-ups. That's it.

The City of Albuquerque has built a par course near our home; it includes a Chin-up station and a Push-up station. When the weather is good, as it almost always is, after Snatches and Squats, I walk down to the par course and do my Chin-ups and

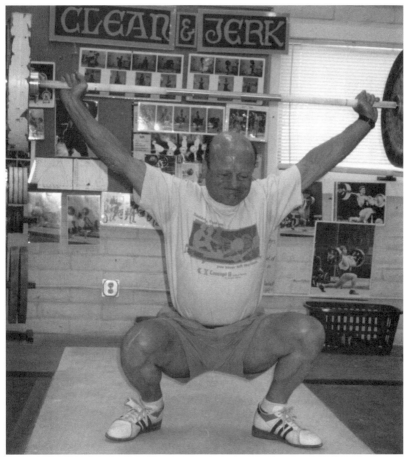

The Squat Snatch is truly acrobatics with a barbell. The bar is pulled slightly above hip level, and then, in a lightning fast move, caught overhead in the full squat position. *Photo by Carl Miller.*

Push-ups. (I do them at home when the weather is nasty or when I'm in a hurry.) Altogether, the Snatches, Squats, Chins and Push-ups, and the walk take about 90 minutes. (I do the crunches at home, before or after the walk.)

This works my whole body pretty well, and it's a nice change of pace. The Push-ups and Chin-ups produce some wonderful soreness in my arms, chest and back. I even get a little sore in the upper abs from the Crunches.

In case you're wondering, workouts A & B are still going well. I haven't noticed any ill effects from repeating workouts every 27 days—rather than every 2 weeks. Everything seems to be progressing just fine.

The journey continues. I'll let you know how it goes.

Now, let's look at some health and longevity issues.

"Health is 50% lifestyle and 10% medicine;
the rest is genetics, environment and luck."
—Arno L. Jensen, M.D.
Cooper Clinic

CHAPTER SIX

Longevity and Health Issues

The Lifestyle Challenge

My friend Arnie Jensen, a physician at the Cooper Clinic in Dallas, Texas, says health is 50% lifestyle and 10% medicine; the rest is largely beyond our control. In other words, we can do five times as much for ourselves as doctors can do for us.

We now have the knowledge to strongly influence our health and longevity. Diet and exercise, two things almost completely within our control, are often the best medicine of all. We have the power. The question is whether we are willing to use it.

Here we discuss things you can do to help yourself live a longer and more productive life. This chapter is about healthy lifestyle. Are you ready to accept the challenge?

Let's start with my responses to two interesting letters. The first deals with hypertension and the second with heart disease and why doctors are often skeptical about lifestyle change.

Self-Help

Dear Clarence: On the advice of my doctor, I took blood pressure medication every day for nine years. No doctor told me to change my diet; no doctor told me to exercise; and no doctor told me that a change of lifestyle might permit me to stop taking medication. Those ideas came to my mind from reading your column and your books.

That was ten years ago. Thanks to your influence, with my doctor's approval, I have been able to stop taking blood pressure medicine. My blood pressure is now normal without any medicine at all.

Thank you for helping me lead a healthier life.

Dear Reader: Congratulations and thank you for the wonderful letter. I am a strong believer in self-help. Many doctors now see that an important part of their role is helping people to help themselves. They acknowledge that lifestyle change is often the most effective medicine of all. You were wise to consult your doctor. No one should stop medication without discussing it with their physician.

Diet, of course, plays a role in the control of blood pressure—obesity and high salt intake are important risk factors—but even more interesting to me is the positive effects of exercise. Dr. Kenneth H. Cooper, founder of the famed Cooper Clinic, says it is now generally accepted that "the more physically fit you are, the less likely you are to suffer from hypertension."

A few years back, I attended a presentation for lawyers at the local medical school by a professor of anatomy who had completed the Boston Marathon only days earlier. A strong runner, he delighted in relating his experience, so I took the opportunity to ask him what effect endurance exercise has on the cardiovascular system. His response was short and to the point. "It makes the whole system stronger," he said.

Endurance exercise opens your arteries. The much publicized autopsy of Clarence DeMar, who was still running marathons at age 70, showed that he had very large coronary arteries, probably developed as a result of his lifetime of vigorous exercise. (A high-resolution CT scan performed at the Cooper Clinic this past year showed that my coronary arteries are "very large" as well.) Regular exercise also opens the large network of tiny blood vessels connecting the arteries with the veins. Both of these factors, larger arteries and more open capillaries, result in lower blood pressure.

It helps to think of your circulatory system as a hose with many branches. Increasing the diameter of the hose reduces the pressure in the system. Likewise, adding hundreds of small connecting tubes or capillaries into which the blood can "escape" reduces the overall pressure. In untrained individuals, the hose is smaller and the connecting branches are constricted or closed, which leads to high blood pressure.

Endurance exercise also makes the heart bigger and stronger so that it can pump more blood with each stroke. That's why well-conditioned athletes have low resting heart rates. Only a fraction of their capacity is required to supply their resting needs. Roger Bannister's resting heart rate was in the 70s before he trained to become the world's first 4-minute miler. At the time of the record, his resting heart rate was less than 40 beats per minute. That means that his resting blood pressure was probably lower as well.

Carol and I use a machine at the su-

Bodybuilders develop the capillary system in each body part they work. The total effect is to enlarge the capillary system all over the body. This allows the blood to spread out, which lowers the overall pressure.

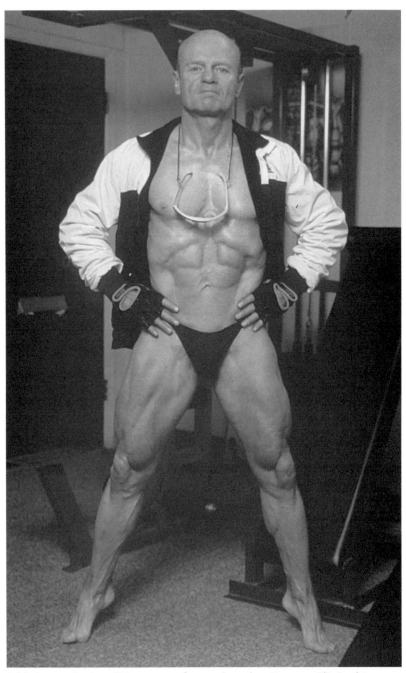

A high-resolution CT scan performed at the Cooper Clinic this past year showed that my coronary arteries are "very large." Carol and I both have youthful blood pressures and resting heart rates under 50. Our active lifestyle is working! *Photo by Pat Berrett.*

permarket where we shop that measures blood pressure and resting heart rate. Stick your arm in the cuff, push a button and the results soon appear. Happily, we both have youthful pressures and resting heart rates under 50. Needless to say, it's reassuring to know that our active lifestyle is working.

To be most effective, exercise should involve a lot of muscle. That's where bodybuilding comes into the blood pressure picture. No other form of exercise systematically trains all the muscles—and blood vessels—like bodybuilding. This is especially true of the upper body muscles which are often neglected in endurance exercises, like running and biking, which involve mainly the lower body. Bodybuilders develop the capillary system in each body part they work. The total effect is to enlarge the capillary system all over the body. This allows the blood to spread out, which lowers the overall pressure.

Weight training is also an effective tool for eliminating unwanted bodyfat. This is very important because being overweight, according to Dr. Cooper, may be the primary factor contributing to hypertension. We don't know exactly how obesity contributes to hypertension, but fat people probably have high blood pressure because the extra weight increases their blood volume and their unused muscles have fewer capillaries. Weight training has the double-barreled effect of expanding the capillary system and also eliminating unwanted bodyfat.

Weight training builds and maintains muscle tissue, and muscle tissue burns calories even at rest. Fat tissue is inactive and burns very few calories. This makes a tremendous difference. Exercise physiologists estimate that one pound of resting muscle burns the equivalent of five pounds of bodyfat over the course of a year.

As you know, self-help requires effort. It won't work if you don't. The benefits come only to those who develop a lifelong exercise habit. Here are two tips to help you stay motivated, one from the endurance side and the other from a strength trainer. Alois Mader, a professor at the German University of Sciences, points out a simple precept of the highly successful Kenyan running program: "[Always] run so that you [will] still enjoy it the next day." Bodybuilding legend Bill Pearl credits a similar approach for his 55-year (and counting) training career. Says Pearl, "It's best to leave a little bit in the gym so you can go back the next day and pick it up and start all over again."

Congratulations again. I hope this additional information encourages you to continue helping yourself. As Lawrence E. Lamb, M.D., wrote not long ago, "Ask not what your doctor can do for you, but what you can do for yourself."

Hold the Scalpel

Dear Clarence: Once a year a general hospital near where I live in Sweden has an open house for the public. I went to listen to a doctor talk about heart disease. To my surprise, not one word was said about the role of lifestyle.

I'd read in one of your books about Dr. Dean Ornish's success in opening clogged arteries with a program of lifestyle change, so when the question and answer session arrived I asked the doctor about the possibility of reversing heart disease through exercise and a very-low-fat diet. I was far from satisfied with his answer. He seemed more interested in heart operations.

Some time ago I talked to a man who was going to have open heart surgery because of clogged coronary arteries. I suggested to him that if he started to take in a diet very low in fat there was a chance he would not need the operation. He wasn't interested. He went into the hospital for the operation and never returned home.

Any comment?

Dear Reader: Your friend's unwillingness to help himself may explain, in part, why the doctor brushed off your question. Many doctors are convinced that an aggressive program of exercise, low-fat diet and stress reduction can reverse heart disease, but they remain skeptical about compliance. This was emphasized in an article on the subject a few years back in *The Physician And Sportsmedicine* and again late last year in *The Wall Street Journal*.

About four years ago, Dean Ornish, M.D. reported in *The Lancet* that his non-surgical, drug-free regimen reduced coronary blockage in most patients in a year and dramatically improved symptoms far sooner. In December of 1998, he published a follow-up report in the *Journal of the American Medical Association* showing even greater reversal of coronary heart disease after five years than after one year.

Patients who followed Dr. Ornish's rigorous diet-and-lifestyle regimen for five years experienced less chest pain and fewer other heart problems than patients who followed the more moderate diet and exercise program recommended by The American Heart Association. The biggest difference between the two programs is that Ornish recommends a strict low-fat (10%), vegetarian diet and the heart group calls for no more than 30 percent of daily calories from fat. Both recommend moderate exercise.

After five years, the coronary arteries were slightly wider in patients on the Ornish program, while those of patients following the Heart Association guidelines were more obstructed.

Ornish's five year report reopened the longstanding debate over the best way to encourage Americans to change their diets and other habits to help prevent heart disease.

Dr. Ornish told *The Wall Street Journal*, "The majority of patients who follow The American Heart Association guidelines got worse and worse, whereas patients who made more extensive changes in diet and lifestyle got better and better."

The heart group's position is that only a small percentage of people could be expected to follow the Ornish regimen.

Retorts Dr. Ornish: "To me the issue isn't what's easy, it's what's true."

"There's no doubt you can slow down the atherosclerotic process and, in the case of many types of lesions, make them much smaller," Dr. Robert W. Wissler, distinguished service professor emeritus of pathology at the University of Chicago, told the *Physician and Sportsmedicine* after the first Ornish report. In addition to the Ornish study, the St. Thomas' Atherosclerosis Regression Study found decreased blockage in 38 percent of patients on a 27%-fat diet. And a German study combining a low-fat, low-cholesterol diet and exercise reported reversal of blockage in 32 percent of patients after one year.

"It's easier for people to make big changes than small ones, even though that's against conventional wisdom."

Ornish says overall adherence to his program was the strongest predictor of improvement, more important than age or disease severity. That's the problem, says *Sportsmedicine*. "Adherence is also the aspect of lifestyle intervention that arouses the most skepticism. Some patients seem to resist cutting fat even to the modest degree advocated by the American Heart Association [30%]." Ornish's answer was the same at one year and five: "It's easier for people to make big changes than small ones, even though that's against conventional wisdom." He says patients who go on the 30%-fat routine have "the worst of both worlds." They feel deprived, and their chest pain isn't improved.

Initially, short-term gains are more important than long-term gains, according to Ornish. On his regimen, angina symptoms generally improve within weeks, even days. "It's a powerful motivator," he says.

The Ornish regimen "will make a lot of people feel better," says Dr. Wissler. "That's what's on his side."

With that background, perhaps you can better understand why the doctor at the open house was not enthusiastic about your question. Let's face it, he's probably had little success motivating people to change their lifestyle. On the other hand, he knows for a fact that surgery works—although it didn't for your acquaintance.

Still, I agree with you—and Dr. Ornish. We should do everything possible to let people know there's a lot they can do to help themselves. It's important to show them that low-fat eating can be enjoyable. The recipes in my books demonstrate that quite convincingly. There's absolutely no need to eat food that doesn't taste good.

Moreover, Dr. Ornish is dead-on when he says that positive feedback is a powerful motivator. The other keys to sticking with a healthy lifestyle are goals, realistic goals—and challenge; when you reach a goal, you must set a new goal.

Surgery often works, but it's risky and expensive. I think you and I agree that a healthy lifestyle is a better alternative. So, hold the scalpel, Doc. Pass the veggies, and show me the way to the gym.

* * * *

Now, let's turn to the serious problem of overfatness, and why weight tables have often given the American people a bum steer.

We'll start with my response to a medical doctor who raised questions about the harmfulness of yo-yo dieting

Yo-Yo Is Not Okay

Dear Clarence: I enclose an article from the *Journal Of The American Medical Association* that reviews the research literature on weight cycling (also called "yo-yo dieting"). The authors conclude that, contrary to conventional wisdom, there is no convincing evidence that this behavior negatively affects metabolism, body composition or overall health. They feel that the studies that do purport to demonstrate such an impact have methodological flaws. They also express concern that obese people not refrain from losing weight because of fear of weight cycling, since the medical and psychological benefits of weight loss really are beyond dispute.

You have written on this subject before and I thought you would be interested in a different perspective.

Keep up the good work.

Dear Doctor: Thanks. I agree that it's useful to challenge assumptions.

The fact that there is so much attention given to weight cycling—the review cites 75 English-language articles—indicates how unsuccessful most people are at keeping weight off. One big problem is that people try too hard. They bite off

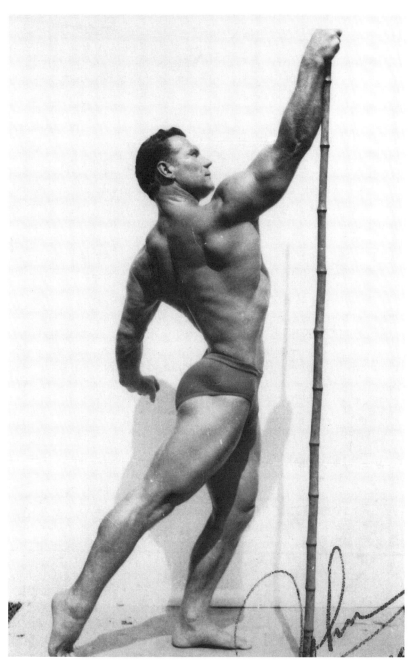

Here's a photo of John Grimek at about 50 years of age. Obviously, John found an exercise regimen that he enjoyed. Grimek continued exercising until shortly before his death last year at 88. *Photo courtesy of the Todd-McLean Collection.*

more than they can chew. They don't see weight control as a lifelong pursuit.

I hope people don't get the idea that yo-yoing has no downside. The literature review didn't find a dearth of evidence that weight cycling has negative effects. Instead, it simply decided the evidence was "not sufficiently compelling." I'm skeptical. At minimum, it seems logical that nature has equipped us to conserve calories with increased efficiency when we are subjected to repeated cycles of feast and famine. That helped us survive in ancient times. Now it just makes yo-yo dieters fatter. Note that the objective of the new report by the National Task Force on the Prevention and Treatment of Obesity was "to address concerns about the effects of weight cycling...." As the report states, at least one review in a professional journal suggested that remaining obese may be healthier than repeated failed attempts to lose weight. The reviewers don't want overweight people to be frightened into giving up. Because, as you say, the benefits of body fat control are beyond dispute.

The critical issue is not whether yo-yo dieting is bad. Of course, it's bad; it signifies repeated failure. The more relevant question is why so many people fail at weight control. As documented by the results of a long-term study conducted by the Federal Centers for Disease Control and Prevention, which you also sent me, the number of Americans who are seriously overweight, after holding steady for 20 years at about a quarter of the population, jumped to 33.4% in the 1988-1991 period. That's an increase of one third! Americans are losing the battle of the bulge big time.

Why? The *JAMA* editorial, which accompanied the study on the prevalence of overweight among U.S. adults, says many things are involved: a plentiful supply of fattening foods, the decline of smoking, genetics, cultural factors and our sedentariness. For most people, however, it boils down to this simple proposition: We eat too much and exercise too little.

Still, dieting per se is not the answer. The recent weight-cycling literature review notwithstanding, alternating between periods of starvation and stuffing just makes things worse. Diets make people uncomfortable and unhappy. Most every diet is followed by an equal and opposite binge. It's far better to adopt a sensible style of eating. We should focus more on the kind of food we eat and less on the amount. If we simply pile on the fruit, vegetables and whole grain products and take it easy on fat and sweets, our natural appetite control mechanism will take care of the rest. We'll never be hungry, and our calories will be under control automatically.

156

Eating a whole-food, low-fat diet is not the complete answer, however. We also need exercise. Controlling body fat level is almost impossible without regular exercise. An exercise regimen of aerobics and weight training works best, but any regular physical activity helps a great deal.

Regardless of the potential benefits, the only exercise program that will work is the one that you are willing to follow. Psychologist Kelly Brownell, Ph.D, head of the Yale University Center for Eating and Weight Disorders and one of the most prolific researchers on yo-yo dieting, says the most important question to ask about exercise is: "Will I be doing this a year from now?" Choose activities you enjoy. Focus on developing a consistent form of activity or set of activities. "It is better for a person to play golf twice a week and walk once a week than to run four miles a day for a week and then stop indefinitely," says Brownell. That's great advice.

> The only diet and exercise program that will work is one that you'll be comfortable with forever. For the great majority, that's the answer to our growing weight problem.

To paraphrase what I said in *The Lean Advantage 2*, the secret to successful weight control—and the solution to the yo-yo problem—boils down to "the comfort factor." The only diet and exercise program that will work is one that you'll be comfortable with forever. For the great majority, that's the answer to our growing weight problem.

Thanks again.

Thin Is Back In

How things change. Fifteen years ago, people asked if I was concerned that maintaining a very low body fat level would shorten my life. Commenting on my near-essential fat level, one fellow wrote: "We both know that 12-15% body fat is necessary for adequate and steady response to day-to-day stress. Getting ripped is great for photos, but it's not a healthy condition to maintain." My response was: "With a common sense approach, ripped looks healthy, feels healthy and *is* healthy."

The proof is in the pudding, as they say. I just attended the 33-year reunion of my law school class. A classmate, a very successful personal injury attorney, delighted me with this comment: "We're all getting older—except for you." After a pause he added, "I looked carefully, and you don't even have any grey in your hair."

Many factors, of course, determine how one ages. Anorexia or

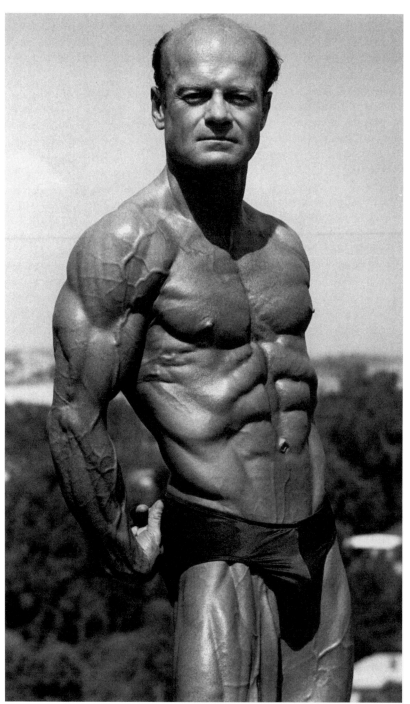

With a common sense approach, ripped looks healthy, feels healthy and is healthy. *Photo by Bill Reynolds.*

extreme dieting carry health risks (I never miss a meal myself), and genetics has a major effect on lifespan. Obviously, I don't have much hair, and the fact that what little I do have isn't white may have no relationship to my low body fat. Be that as it may, the scientific community is coming around to my "lean for life" philosophy. A recent study of middle-aged men by the Harvard School of Public Health found that the leaner a man is, the longer he's likely to live.

The research contradicts a decades-long trend that I've criticized before. Height/weight tables have been revised upward; physicians, insurers and the government have allowed increasingly heavier men and women to be categorized as healthy. New health-based weight criteria were issued suggesting that a 10 or 15 pound gain after age 34 is acceptable.

"The recommended weights keep going up, which is almost like an endorsement from the government that you can keep eating more and getting larger," I-Min Lee, the Harvard School of Public Health epidemiologist who led the latest research, told the *Washington Post*. The trend has been driven, she said, by badly designed studies that have found death rates to be highest not only among the fattest but also among the thinnest people studied, with lifespans longest in the middle ranges. Most importantly, they failed to "control" for smokers, who often are thin and tend to die earlier. Including them in the studies bias the results in favor of weighing a few pounds more.

Reversing this trend, the Harvard study finds that, all other things being equal, leaner is better. The researchers propose no lower limit for men *as long as they are healthy*.

The research, part of an ongoing study of Harvard Alumni, tracked the medical fates of more than 19,000 men who were, on average, 47 years old when the study began in 1962. They found that the thinnest 20% of the men were about 40% less likely to have died by 1988 than were the heaviest 20%. Even more significant, according to the researchers, men in the thinnest fifth were 60% less likely to die from heart disease than were their heaviest counterparts.

Of particular importance to me and others who train, Harvard's Lee said that even though the study collected little data on caloric intake there was some evidence that the leanest individuals ate more than the heaviest, but maintained their low weight by being more active.

"Although it is common for most 'normal' adults to grow fatter as they age, those who engage in heavy resistance training increase their lean body mass *and decrease body fat*."

159

"Go ahead and eat," she said, "but you have to get out and exercise more."

Bodybuilders may be the best exemplars of Lee's point; they eat a lot and exercise a lot. The latest edition of *Exercise Physiology* by Drs. William D. McArdle, Frank I. Katch and Victor L. Katch (Williams & Wilkins, 1996) emphasizes the importance of weight training in controlling body fat, especially as we age. Say the authors, "Although it is common for most 'normal' adults to grow fatter as they age, those who engage in heavy resistance training increase their lean body mass *and decrease body fat.*" (emphasis added) Using photos of Bill Pearl at 37 and 59 as verification, the authors conclude: "Individuals who engage in resistance training seem to defy certain aspects of the typical aging process." Waneen W. Spirduso, Ed.D, makes basically the same point in *Physical Dimensions of Aging* (Human Kinetics, 1995), using as evidence photos of your author at *15, 31, 43 and 55.*

That brings to mind a general criticism I have of national health guidelines. They cater to the lowest common denominator. They assume that people are not willing to do what is really best for them. For example, they know that we would be leaner and healthier, and probably live longer, if we consumed 20% or less of our calories in fat. Nevertheless, 30% is recommended. I believe that's because the government doesn't think people will cut fat intake as much as they really should.

That attitude, of course, is at work in the weight tables which say it's OK to gain weight (fat) as we age. It's operative in current activity and exercise guidelines as well. The experts behind government recommendations know that many people have a hard time sticking to an exercise program, so they emphasize that any activity is better than nothing. That's true, of course, but it's hardly the ideal approach.

My friend, health behavior psychologist Richard A. Winett, Ph.D., made essentially the same point in a letter to the *New York Times* and in his *Master Trainer* newsletter. He questioned the trend to emphasize total calories expended over intensity of effort. Every serious bodybuilder knows that intensity and progression are the key ingredients in productive training. Nevertheless, Winett observed that in response to disappointing adherence outcomes in the past, health guidelines have focused on duration and frequency in exercise and de-emphasized intensity. They settle for any activity that burns extra calories. Winett believes this does the public a disservice.

For example, five hours weekly of cutting the grass or some similar activity burns about 1500 calories. But the benefits are

160

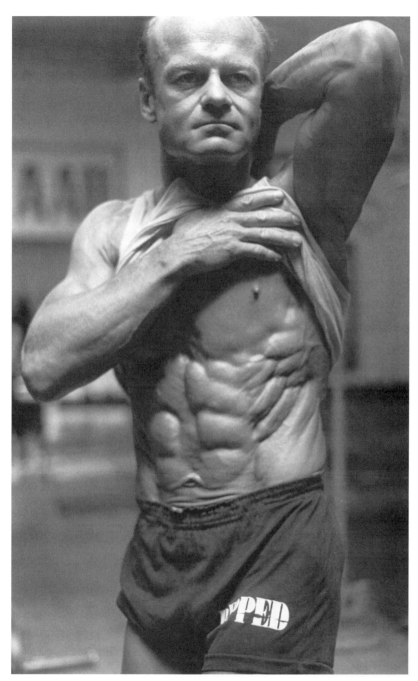

The scientific community is coming around to my "lean for life" philosophy. *This photo by Bill Reynolds* shows me at my leanest.

negligible compared to two 30-minute sessions of high-intensity exercise each week walking uphill on a treadmill culminating in a near maximum heart rate—burning less than 600 calories. Cutting the grass burns more calories but the treadmill workout, with it's low-frequency, low-volume and high-intensity, produces a much higher level of fitness. Moreover, according to Winett, research shows that as previously unfit men become fitter, their death rates decreased 7.9% for each minute longer they could walk during a standard treadmill test in which the angle of incline increases each minute. In other words, fitness and longevity increase together.

> "To fall into the trap of convincing people they can get great benefit from very little effort and commitment is neither good science or public policy."

I agree with Dick Winett: "To fall into the trap of convincing people they can get great benefit from very little effort and commitment is neither good science or public policy."

New Federal Weight Guidelines

On June 17, 1998 the National Heart, Lung, and Blood Institute announced new guidelines defining healthy and unhealthy body weights. The first height-weight tables were established by the Metropolitan Life Insurance Company in the 1950s; Americans have gotten fatter every decade since, with more than a third now classified as obese. According to the latest numbers, fully 55 percent are overweight!

Although the new guidelines are meant to encourage doctors to monitor and treat weight problems as regularly as cholesterol and blood pressure, I'm dubious that they will be any more effective than the earlier charts. Nevertheless, the authorities are moving in the right direction by warning an additional 29 million Americans that their weight may be a problem. In the face of the alarming increase in the number of Americans in the overweight and obese categories, the new federal guidelines reverse the previous trend discussed in the last section. At least they are no longer telling people that weight gain with age is okay—because everybody does it.

The new numbers are age and gender neutral. All you need to determine where you stand is your body-mass index, or BMI. BMI is a single number representing your height and weight. A BMI of 24 or under is said to be consistent with good health; from 25 to 29 is overweight; and 30 or above is obese and cause for major concern. People with a BMI from 25 to 27 are borderline risk, but BMIs above 27, and especially above 30 are clearly associated with a greater incidence of diabetes, stroke, heart disease, some cancers and other ills.

Interestingly, at 5' 6" and 155 pounds I'm on the cusp of the overweight category. (The guidelines do acknowledge that some very muscular people may have a high BMI without health risk.) The formula is 703 x weight in pounds, divided by height in inches squared. Do the numbers and you'll see that my BMI is 25 (703 x 155 = 108,965 divided by 66 x 66 or 4356, is 25).

> **Most people don't need to calculate their BMI to know whether they are too fat. It's simple. Just take off your clothes and look in the mirror.**

Obviously, BMI is only a ballpark figure, as the guidelines recognize. They emphasize that waist measurement is a good check on BMI. With a waist measurement of only 30 inches, I'd clearly get a clean bill of health. But people with lots of upper body fat and a "pear" shape are at risk, no matter what their BMI score.

Most people don't need to calculate their BMI to know whether they are too fat. It's simple. Just take off your clothes and look in the mirror.

Now that we know Americans are in the midst of a fat epidemic, let's look at a weight control method that required no help from doctors or the government.

Fat Loss Mother Nature's Way

As we just noted, more and more Americans are getting fat. In fact, current trends predict that all Americans will be obese by 2230. Obviously, we desperately need a solution for the problem of creeping obesity.

Well, we don't have to wait another day. Our bodies, with a few rare exceptions, already have a marvelous ability to balance calorie intake and expenditure. All we have to do is start working with—rather than against—our biology. It takes a little longer, but the payoff for most people is permanent leanness.

Few of us get fat fast. We get fat very slowly. According to *Physiology of Sport and Exercise*, the beautifully designed textbook by Jack H. Wilmore and David L. Costill (Human Kinetics, 1994), the average person in this country will gain approximately one pound each year after age 25, or a total of 30 pounds of excess weight by age 55. But that's not the whole story. We also lose a half pound of muscle each year due to lack of exercise. That means the average person actually gains 1.5 pounds of fat each year, or 45 pounds of fat over 30 years. Wow, you might think, that sounds unrelenting, even a little scary.

To the contrary, considered day by day, it's not at all insurmountable. In fact, it's quite manageable. The average gain of 1.5 pounds of fat represents an excess of only 5,250 calories per year (one pound of fat contains 3,500 calories). That's less than 15 calories per day or, as Wilmore and Costill observe, the amount found in one potato chip. In other words, even the average sedentary person comes within one potato chip each day of energy balance.

The body's ability to balance energy intake and expenditure to such a remarkable degree has led scientists to propose that bodyweight is regulated similar to the way in which body temperature is regulated. Wilmore and Costill say there is excellent evidence that the body adapts to major changes in calorie intake by altering the metabolism. When we go on a very low calorie diet, our metabolism slows down to conserve energy. Conversely, when we overeat our metabolism speeds up to "waste" the surplus calories.

> "There is probably no biological reason why men and women [should] get fatter as they age."

Think about that! Even in this age of fast food and automation, our body's natural balancing mechanism brings us within a hair's breadth of weight equilibrium. McArdle, Katch and Katch, authors of the textbook referred to earlier, reinforce this point with an important corollary: "There is probably no biological reason why men and women [should] get fatter as they age," they assert. In short, if we just help the system a little each day we can achieve absolute balance, and by tweaking it a little more we can create a negative balance—and lose fat. Here's some general principles to keep in mind.

As noted, our metabolism slows in response to severe calorie restriction. Robert Robergs, Ph.D., who did his doctoral work in exercise physiology under Dr. Costill at Ball State University, Muncie, Indiana, and who is now director of the Center for Exercise at the University of New Mexico, says the metabolism slowdown can be as much as 500 calories per day after six weeks on a very low calorie diet. "That's a huge problem," he emphasizes. "It makes it harder and harder for people to lose weight."

That's why Arno L. Jensen, M.D., my friend who practices preventive medicine and radiology at the Cooper Clinic, urges his patients to lose slowly, not more than one half to one pound a week. To convince them Dr. Jensen uses a model of five pounds of fat. "That shocks them," he says, because they don't realize

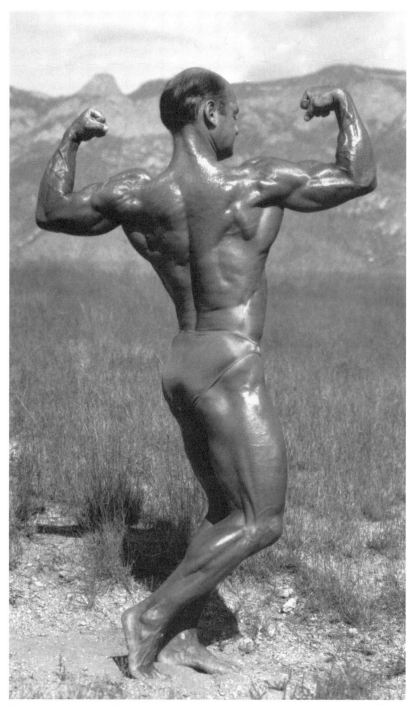

People who exercise have an easier time balancing calories. *Photo by Guy Appelman*.

how much flesh five pounds of fat represents. He shows them that model and says, "You can lose five of these in a year's time by losing [only] a half pound a week." "That just really motivates them" to lose slowly. "That makes them feel good," Jensen adds, because people dread severe dieting.

It's common knowledge, of course, that rapid weight losses are usually temporary. A slowed metabolism is one reason why the weight is soon regained. Another reason, according to Wilmore and Costill, is that rapid losses are often mostly water. The body has built-in safety mechanisms to prevent an imbalance in body fluid levels, so the lost water is eventually replaced.

Similarly, it's not a good idea to limit the quantity of food you eat. Forcing yourself to stop eating before you're full and satisfied doesn't work very well. My observation is that few people can do it for long, and it's not necessary anyway. As explained earlier in this book, eating a balanced diet low in fat and high in natural carbohydrates will usually do the trick. G. Ken Goodrick, Ph.D., an associate professor of medicine at Baylor College of Medicine in Houston and an expert on weight control, agrees that a diet low in fat and high in fiber is best, "because it is easier to eat fewer calories without having to eat small portions." You don't have to worry about restricting the amount you eat, because you become full before exceeding your calorie needs. Your body's appetite control mechanism tells you when you've had enough.

Dr. Jenson cautions, however, that you must focus on the whole diet, and not just low fat. "America is getting fat eating a low fat diet," he maintains. "People are keen on eating a low fat diet, but forget that low fat diets have calories." Like Dr. Goodrick, Jensen urges eating plenty of bulky and filling—but low calorie—whole grains and cereals, fruits and vegetables.

A sedentary lifestyle throws the appetite off, causing us to eat more calories than we expend.

Everybody knows that exercise burns calories and speeds up the metabolism, but less well known is its appetite curbing effect. Exercise facilitates the body's natural regulatory ability. This was first demonstrated in 1954 by world-famous nutritionist Jean Mayer. He reported that animals exercising for periods of 20 minutes to one hour per day ate less than non-exercising animals. He concluded from this and other studies that when activity falls below a certain minimum level, food intake does not drop a like amount—and fat begins to accumulate. Apparently, this is one reason why the average person gains fat every year. A sedentary lifestyle throws the appetite off, causing us to eat more calories than we expend. That's not to say that lumberjacks, marathoners, bodybuilders and other very active people eat less than sedentary individuals. They eat more, of course. The difference is that people who exercise have an easier time balancing calories. Dr. Robergs notes, for example, that Tour de France cyclists maintain or lose weight consuming more than 5000 calories a day.

Now, let's end with an activity that doesn't live up to it's billing. (We discussed this point earlier, but it's so widely misunderstood that it bears repeating.)

According to Wilmore and Costill, low-intensity aerobic exercise does *not* necessarily burn more fat than high-intensity aerobic exercise. It's true that the body uses a higher proportion of fat for energy at lower exercise intensities. However, total calories expended are greater during high-intensity aerobics—and the fat burned is the same. For example, an average 40-year-old male will burn the same number of calories from fat exercising for 30 minutes at 50 percent of capacity and at 75 percent. He burns about 145 calories of fat in both cases. Importantly, however, during the higher intensity workout he expends approximately 50 percent more total calories, about 435 compared to only 290 in the course of the low-intensity session.

Dr. Robergs isn't sure how the fat burn fallacy got started, but he believes that people simply like the word "easy." He thinks they grab on to the idea, because it makes easy training "more readily acceptable." Nevertheless, he says, "you can't convert a relative contribution to an absolute value; it's the total amount of calories [burned] that's most important."

"There is another issue too," Robergs adds, which makes the intensity of the workout important for fat loss. A more intense approach, he explains, "is more conducive to improving the muscle's ability to use fat." The more fit you become, the more likely you are to use fat as fuel. "When you become more fit you are just better able to metabolize fat for any given activity you do," Robergs stresses. In other words, you burn more fat 24 hours a day.

Give Mother Nature's weight control a try. It works. I guarantee it.

Next, let's look at my response to a man who was concerned about getting too much of a good thing.

Overtraining May Be Deadly

Dear Clarence: At 76, I still lift for an hour or so four times a week, and I feel great. I also do some hand balancing.

My reason for writing is to get your comments on Ken Cooper's book warning of the dangers of doing too much exercise. It's a bit scary. We have people like Bob Hope and George Burns who never lifted anything but a cigar and they aged very well. It makes you wonder. Nevertheless, I plan to stay in shape with exercise as long as I can.

Dear Reader: I understand your concern. Dr. Kenneth H. Cooper's *Anti-Oxidant Revolution* says excessive exercise may well kill you. That's startling coming from the man whose 1968 book *Aerobics* is credited with starting the jogging boom. The focus of Cooper's book is research suggesting that excessive, high-intensity exercise may produce enough free radicals to create serious health problems. As you may know, free radicals are unstable oxygen molecules produced by the body. They can damage things (other chemicals and cellular structures) they come in contact with and have been linked to health problems including cancer, heart disease, premature aging and cataracts. The key word is "excessive." When you read the details, it becomes clear that Dr. Cooper hasn't turned thumbs down on exercise. Well into his 60s, Cooper himself still runs hard. What's more, he encourages weight training.

Dr. Cooper's conclusion that there may be a link between overtraining and disease is based on both clinical observations and research. In particular, he has become alarmed at the increased frequency of irregular heartbeat found in highly conditioned runners who have been exercising for many years. He is also bothered by the frequency of prostate cancer among older marathoners and "ultra" athletes. Cooper's concern finds support in the study of Harvard alumni by Stanford University's Ralph Paffenbarger, M.D.

Cooper's theory is that moderate exercise protects us against free radical damage but overtraining, "distress" type of training, may actually increase the risk of free radical damage— and research seems to bear that out.

Paffenbarger found that death rates were lower for men who were involved in regular physical activity. The death rates declined steadily as the number of calories burned in regular physical activity increased—but only up to a point. Death rates began to go up slightly among men expending more than 3000 calories per week. Epidemiologists refer to this as the "reverse J-slope phenomenon," because of the way it looks on a graph. The death rate slopes down as exercise goes up, but at the highest level of exercise the line suddenly turns back up, like the tail of a reverse "J." Exercise helps, but it can turn around and bite you.

Cooper's theory is that moderate exercise protects us against free radical damage but overtraining, "distress" type of training, may actually increase the risk of free radical damage—and research seems to bear that out. One 1988 study on ultra marathoners, who raced for 50 miles, revealed increases in free radical damage; whereas, runners who completed the half marathon (13.1 miles) experienced no measurable free radical damage.

A 1993 study at Cooper's own Institute for Aerobic Research compared free radical production in 10 highly trained men and women and 10 sedentary men and women. The trained men had been running an average of 22 miles per week and the trained women were running an average of 10 miles. Somewhat surprisingly, the trained women had the lowest level of free radical activity. The trained males, who ran twice as much as the women, had the highest level. The untrained men and women fell in the middle.

So what does Dr. Cooper recommend? What does he do himself?

First, Cooper says exercise bolsters the body's natural defenses against free radicals. He recommends what he calls "lower-inten-

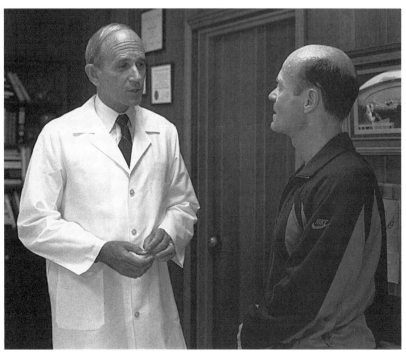

Dr. Ken Cooper and I compare treadmill times. Well into his 60s, Cooper still runs hard and look great. *Photo by Justin Joseph.*

sity" endurance exercise at 65% to 80% of your heart rate maximum. For health and longevity fitness, he suggests two miles of fast walking three times a week or its equivalent. In addition, he believes that strength training is essential for good health, especially as we grow older. He suggests training with weights for 20 or 30 minutes two or three times a week on alternate days from endurance sessions. He recommends 8-12 reps and gradual poundage increases to avoid soreness and injury, which he says are signs of free radical damage. Above all, he says: "Do not push yourself to do frequent, high-intensity exercise, particularly to the point of total exhaustion and chronic fatigue."

Tellingly, Cooper himself is not satisfied with health and longevity fitness. He strives for what he terms an "athletic level of fitness—which does not involve overtraining." Using the new fitness point system introduced in this book, Cooper says that requires only 35-points a week: the equivalent of running two miles in less than 20 minutes, four times per week, or walking three miles in less than 45 minutes, fives times per week.

Cooper, however, continues to earn 50- to 75-points per week, because "that is the level at which I feel the best!" He finds it's easier to stay motivated at that level. I agree: Training is boring if you don't challenge yourself.

Finally—and this is what's really new from Cooper—he has gone from opposing vitamins supplements in any amount to recommending daily megadoses of the antioxidants: Vitamin E, Vitamin C and beta carotene. Antioxidant supplements, he says, are essential, especially if you are training at the athletic fitness level. (I hope he's right, because I've been taking vitamin and mineral supplements since I was a child; in addition to a complete multi-vitamin-mineral formulation, I take extra vitamin C and E every day.)

> **In a nutshell, Dr. Cooper is simply counseling moderation. That's always been good advice.**

Feel better now? You should. Anyone still hand balancing at 76 is doing something right. Training for an hour four times a week, as you do, seems to fit Cooper's guidelines nicely. I train only twice a week, one day of aerobics and one of lifting, but my intensity level is very high. If I was you, I wouldn't change a thing.

In a nutshell, Dr. Cooper is simply counseling moderation. That's always been good advice.

(For those interested in a technical discussion of overtraining and its ramifications, I recommend *Overtraining in Sport* edited by Richard B. Kreider, Ph.D, Andrew L. Fry, Ph.D., and Mary L. O'Toole, Ph.D. (Human Kinetics, 1997).)

* * * *

We'll shift gears again at this point and discuss two new health-related issues, both of which have affected me personally. The first deals with a condition that may play a critical role in destroying our arteries. Happily, it appears to respond to nothing more demanding than taking a few vitamins.

What's Your Homocysteine?

Homocysteine? Like many doctors, I never heard of it—until the Cooper Clinic's Dr. Arno Jensen told me mine is normal, but higher than he recommends.

Homocysteine (pronounced HO-mo-SIS-teen) is an amino acid that attacks the lining of our arteries setting off a chain of events that often leads to heart attack or stroke. The startling fact is that people with none of the commonly known risk factors (sedentary lifestyle, smoking, obesity, high blood pressure, high cholesterol) often have high levels of homocysteine in their blood. What's more, about a fourth of all heart attacks occur in people with normal cholesterol and none of the other health hazards. That's why homocysteine has been called the "silent killer."

> Homocysteine (pronounced HO-mo-SIS-teen) is an amino acid that attacks the lining of our arteries setting off a chain of events that often leads to heart attack or stroke.

As long ago as the late '60s, Dr. Kilmer McCully began to suspect a link between homocysteine and arterial disease, but until recently most doctors were too focused on cholesterol to pay much attention. McCully discovered the connection while studying a rare genetic disorder called homocystinuria. Children born with this condition lack proper levels of an enzyme required to process homocysteine, so it reaches extremely high levels in their blood. If untreated, they often die of heart attack or stoke before reaching adulthood.

McCully observed during autopsy that the victim's arteries were scarred and thickened like those of elderly heart patients. If high levels of homocysteine can destroy young arteries, he reasoned, then lower levels over a long period of time might cause vascular disease in adults. As I'll explain shortly, subsequent research strongly suggests that McCully's hunch was correct.

Like cholesterol, homocysteine performs a desirable function. It is derived from the essential amino acid methionine and is used to build and maintain tissue. During normal conditions excess homocysteine—with the help of some B-complex vitamins—is converted back to methionine or broken down for excretion. Understanding the damage done when the conversion process fails helps clarify the harmful role of cholesterol. Dr. McCully believes homocysteine buildup is "the underlying cause of heart disease."

Arterial disease usually develops over a long period of time; the process, if not the root cause, is well known. It begins when something injures the lining of the artery and the body tries to repair the damage. In simplified terms, scar tissue builds up, like it would on other parts of the body, inhibiting blood flow and promoting the formation of clots.

Many people probably assume that cholesterol in the blood somehow causes the initial injury to the arterial wall. Dr. McCully says that's not so, that the first injury is caused by excessive homocysteine. The injury makes the blood vessels vulnerable to cholesterol buildup; the scaring and thickening on the arterial wall gives the cholesterol a place to stick and grow.

Significantly, smoking tends to raise homocysteine levels. Homocysteine levels also increase in old age. And when arterial disease runs in families there is often a minor genetically based flaw in homocysteine metabolism; roughly one person in eight inherits a gene that slows disposal of excess homocysteine. (That may be my problem. My father had arterial disease. I don't know about his homocysteine level, but he battled high cholesterol for years. He died from a stroke.)

Dr. McCully's hypothesis is still based on circumstantial evidence, but vindicating his long-held belief, *Newsweek* reported in a cover story: "An avalanche of new studies suggest that... homocysteine plays a critical role in destroying our arteries." (It should be noted that one recent study published in *Circulation* challenged those studies, finding no link between homocysteine and heart disease.)

As is usually the case, the evidence starts outside the human body. In test-tube studies, homocysteine not only injures blood-vessel linings but accelerates the buildup of scar tissue and promotes the formation of blood clots. Moreover, researchers have long known that homocysteine injections produce arterial plaques in animals.

"Homocysteine appears to respond to nothing more demanding than eating more vegetables and taking a few vitamins."

People studies also provide convincing evidence. Harvard researchers followed 14,000 male physicians for five years and found those with homocysteine levels in the highest 5% had three times the heart attack risk of those in the bottom 90%. Likewise, researchers involved in the famous Framingham Heart Study found that people with high homocysteine levels are the most likely to suffer from dangerous narrowing of the carotid artery, the main vessel feeding blood to the brain. And Norwegian scientists, in a study involving 21,000 men and women, showed that heart patients with elevated homocysteine are the most likely to die.

So how can homocysteine be controlled? Surprisingly, and unlike cholesterol, the solution appears to be simple and inexpensive. *Time* magazine reported: "Homocysteine appears to respond to nothing more demanding than eating more vegetables and taking a few vitamins."

Recall that B-complex vitamins help breakdown homocysteine. It stands to reason, therefore, that a lack of key B vitamins would "freeze" homocysteine metabolism, allowing the substance to accumulate in the bloodstream and damage blood vessels. It also seems logical that supplying more B vitamins would help the body to reduce homocysteine to safe levels. That seems to be how it works. Simply consuming more vitamin B6, B12 and folic acid could be all that's required to disarm homocysteine.

Two large studies directly correlate folic acid and B6 with vascular disease. The first study, reported in a recent issue of the *Journal of the American Medical Association*, was part of the ongoing Nurses' Health Study. Researchers followed more than 80,000 women without heart disease for 14 years. Those least likely to have a heart attack consumed more than 400 mcg. (micrograms or one thousandth of a milligram) of folic acid a day from food or supplements. Likewise, those who consumed more than 4 milligrams of Vitamin B6 a day had the lowest heart disease rates.

The second study was published in *Circulation*. Researchers measured levels of folate and vitamin B6 in the blood of 800 healthy volunteers and 750 people with vascular disease. They also measured homocysteine. Patients with vascular disease had high homocysteine levels compared with the healthy volunteers. In men—but not women—with vascular disease, high homocysteine went hand-in-hand with low folate levels. People with vascular disease also had low B6 levels, even though many did not have high homocysteine.

Many physicians now recommend that everyone get at least 400 mcg of folate a day.

That's pretty strong evidence. Even though we are still waiting for a controlled study, where some people are given vitamins and others a dummy pill, showing that supplements reduce the incidents of heart attack and stroke, many physicians now recommend that everyone get at least 400 mcg of folate a day.

That amount was found to be most protective against heart disease in the latest results from the Nurses' Health Study. (Those with a flawed homocysteine metabolism may require more than 400 mcg. I'll discuss Dr. Jensen's advice to me in a moment.)

Why the emphasis on folic acid? Unless you're a strict vegetarian, chances are you're getting plenty of B12. Vitamin B6 is also easy to come by, since it's added to many processed foods. But folic acid is another story. Folate is found mostly in beans, grains and greens, which are hardly abundant in the normal American diet. Nearly half of Americans get less than 200 mcg, the current FDA for men, and only a small minority get 400 mcg.

In my own case, blood drawn in the course of my latest exam at the Cooper Clinic showed my homocysteine to be 11.2 umol/L, at the upper end of the 8-12 normal range. (Between 12 and 15 is borderline, and over 15 is considered high risk.)

My result sounds OK, and Dr. Jensen says it's not a reason for major concern. Still, there's a problem: The risk for vascular disease increases progressively with homocysteine concentrations above 9. Ideally, Dr. Jensen says he'd like to see mine below 9. (That may be especially important in view of my family history of vascular disease.)

My diet is already excellent. Unlike most Americans, I eat plenty of grains, greens and beans. Computer analysis (excluding supplements) shows that my intake of all the B vitamins is well above recommended levels. For example, my folic acid intake is 912 mcg, more than 4 times the RDA. In addition, I take a multi vitamin/mineral packet containing all the B complex vitamins. I am already meeting the Cooper Clinic recommendations for heavy exercisers over 50 (men and women): folic acid 800 mcg, B6 50 mg and B12 400 mcg. What should I do?

As indicated earlier, it is possible that I am among the one in eight people who have inherited a flawed gene that slows the disposal of homocysteine. To test that possibility doctors often recommend a daily multivitamin containing 400 mcg of folic acid plus an additional 800 mcg. If that doesn't bring the homocysteine level down in 8 weeks, the dosage may be increased to 2 mg/day for another 8 weeks. Folic acid supplements are considered safe up to 5 mg/day.

It took two tries, but the usual prescription worked for me. First, I upped my supplemental folic acid intake to 1200 mcg, based on Dr. Jensen's advice. Allowing time for the change to work, I had my blood tested again in two months. That helped; the test showed progress. My homocysteine dropped to 10, an improvement of 11 percent, but still above 9, where the risk begins to rise. Again on Dr. Jensen's advice, I increased my folic

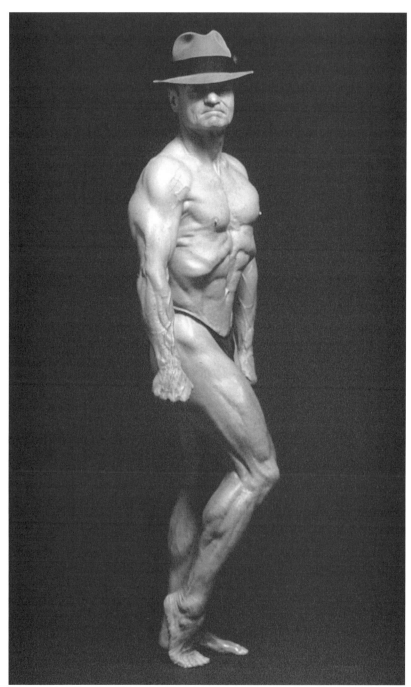

I eat plenty of grains, greens and beans, but I may be among the one in eight people who have inherited a flawed gene that slows the disposal of homocysteine. *Photo by Pat Berrett.*

acid to 3200 mcg. I also added 1000 mcg. of vitamin B12. That did it. My third test showed that my homocysteine had dropped to 7.9, well under the critical 9.0 level that Dr. Jensen targets.

I will maintain my current level of folate and B12 supplementation, and continue taking the multiple vitamin/mineral packet that I've taken for years. I'll continue to have my blood tested regularly, of course.

Needless to say, I'm thankful that Dr. Jensen and the Cooper Clinic alerted me to this newly prominent risk factor, the big one that may be the underlying cause of vascular disease.

It is indeed gratifying to see that we can help ourselves in matters of this kind. As Dr. Jensen often says, our health is largely in our own hands.

What's your homocysteine level?

Now, as promised in chapter two, let's talk about the health benefits of certain dietary fats.

Add a Little "Good Fat"

I added a little fat to my diet for a good reason, and discovered a far better reason for doing so: My total cholesterol/HDL ratio improved from "very good" to "excellent". Even better, my triglycerides dropped 50 percent. What's more, the added fat may have helped me become leaner.

Recent evidence strengthens the connection between high triglycerides and heart disease.

Triglycerides are the fats that circulate in the blood. They are formed in the liver from the fats you eat or from the body's own synthesis of fat. They're essential for good health; your tissues rely on triglycerides for energy. But like cholesterol, when elevated they are implicated in arterial disease.

The importance of triglycerides has been a subject of some debate, but recent evidence strengthens the connection between high triglycerides and heart disease. The New England Journal of Medicine *Health News* recently highlighted a Danish study involving 3000 healthy men. This study, called the Copenhagen Male Study, found that the risk of having a first heart attack was twice as high in those with the highest triglyceride levels as in those with the lowest levels.

Triglyceride levels can range over 1000 (over 5000 in extreme cases), but the Danish study found that the risk of heart attack substantially rose at levels above 140. Most doctors consider 100 or less ideal.

My medical and fitness exams at the Cooper Clinic over the

last ten years have consistently shown my cholesterol profile to be very good. On the first visit, in 1988, my cholesterol was normal at 216 and my total cholesterol/HDL risk ratio was 3.7 (normal is 5.0 and below 4.0 is considered very good). My triglycerides, however, have always been slightly elevated. In 1988, they were 153, slightly above the normal range of 40-150. The pattern was the same in subsequent visits: My cholesterol ranged up to 228 (1992) and my triglycerides were 157 and 155 in 1989 and 1992, respectively.

Something happened in 1998, however.

My cholesterol dropped to 197—most doctors like to see cholesterol below 200—moving my cholesterol/HDL ratio into the excellent category, at 3.3; my HDL cholesterol, the good kind, remained in the excellent category, at 60. That means my risk of having a heart attack is now less than one-half the average. The really good news, however, was that my triglycerides plummeted to 95. On a retest eight weeks later, they dropped another 20 percent, to 76.

The reason my triglycerides dropped from borderline risk to ideal, I believe, was a seemingly minor change in my diet about six months earlier. For more than 20 years I've eaten a low fat, medium protein, high complex-carbohydrate diet. I've also exercised regularly, both weight training and aerobics. That was no different. I made only one change.

> My research suggests the addition of only a little over one tablespoon of oil caused the small, but significant improvement in my cholesterol—and the profound reduction in my blood triglycerides.

To make my meals stay with me a little longer, I added 1/2 teaspoon of vegetable oil (first olive and then flax seed) to each of my meals and snacks. This was done to take advantage of the fact that fat leaves the stomach slowly, which delays the return of hunger. It worked pretty well; I did feel satisfied longer. More importantly, however, my research suggests the addition of only a little over one tablespoon of oil caused the small, but significant improvement in my cholesterol—and the profound reduction in my blood triglycerides.

Everyone agrees that some dietary fat is necessary for good health. In *The Lean Advantage*, published in 1984, I pointed out the need for the essential fatty acids found in nuts, seeds, grains and other foods, and cautioned bodybuilders against trying to completely eliminate fat from their diet. Agreement breaks down, however, on how much dietary fat is ideal.

Low-fat advocate and strict vegetarian John A. McDougall, M.D., author of many books and director of the McDougall Pro-

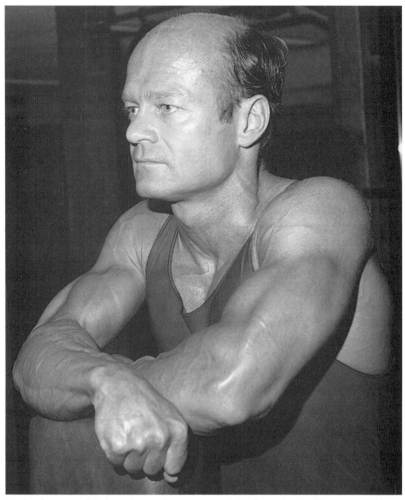

It made me think twice when a seemingly minor dietary change caused my cholesterol to drop 25 percent and cut my triglycerides in half. *Photo by Bill Reynolds.*

gram at St. Helena Hospital in the Napa Valley of California, wrote in *The McDougall Program For A Healthy Heart* (Plume, 1996): "Since all foods contain fat, you cannot create a diet composed of whole foods that's inadequate in fat. It can't be done."

Dean Ornish, M.D., whose ground breaking Lifestyle Heart Trial reversing coronary artery blockage was discussed earlier in this chapter, is also in the very-low fat camp.

On the other hand, Artemis P. Simopoulos, M.D., president of The Center For Genetics, Nutrition and Health in Washington, D.C. and for nine consecutive years chairperson of the Nutrition Coordinating Committee of the National Institutes of Health, says a diet high in "good fats" (monounsaturated and polyunsaturated) is the key to optimum health. In *The Omega Plan* (Harper Collins, 1998), she recommends eating 30-35 percent of your calories as fat (mostly "good fats").

Dr. Simopoulos says new research shows that eating a very low-fat diet "turns your body into a fat-making machine!" According to Simopoulos, it's one of our built-in survival mechanisms. Sensing that a fat famine is under way, the body converts carbohydrates into fat that circulate in your blood as triglycerides. On a high fat diet, however, the body says, "Okay, I'm getting an adequate supply of fats in my diet, so I don't need to make any of my own."

Actually, it's well known that a low-fat, high-carbohydrate diet can drive up triglycerides. This mainly occurs when calorie consumption is excessive, however. A study conducted by Ernst J. Schaefer, M.D., and his colleagues at the Lipid Metabolism Laboratory at Tufts University School of Medicine and reported in the *Journal of the American Medical Association* demonstrated that eating bulky, high-fiber foods usually solves the problem.

The study compared the effect of eating the average US diet, which contains 35% fat, with a high-bulk, high-fiber diet containing 15 percent fat. In addition to fat content, the critical difference was that the high-fiber diet took up more room in the stomach; it weighed 30% more than the diet most Americans eat. In fact, when required to eat enough of the bulky diet to maintain bodyweight the "subjects frequently complained...of abdominal fullness and satiety before the end of the meals." In a final phase, where they were allowed to eat as much as they wanted, Dr. Schaefer said the "patients all adjusted downward." Importantly, when given a choice, they automatically ate less — and lost weight.

The fear that a low-fat, high-carbohydrate diet can increase triglycerides proved well founded, but only when the subjects were forced to eat enough calories to maintain weight. Triglycerides increased 47.3% compared to the level on the average diet.

Happily, when the participants adjusted their intake of the bulky, low-fat diet to suit themselves, the outcome was much more positive. Not only did they lose weight, their LDL cholesterol (the bad kind) declined 24.3%. Significantly, when the subjects ate only as much as they wanted, their triglycerides did not go up.The message from Dr. Schaefer's study is clear: Stick to a bulky, whole foods, low-fat diet. You'll be leaner, because you'll be satisfied eating fewer calories. And your triglycerides will be fine.

Okay, but I eat a bulky, high-fiber, low-fat diet. What happened to me?

Heredity plays a large role in these matters. Dr. Jensen believes that may be my problem. My father had diabetes and heart trouble, and I probably have a genetic predisposition in the direction of high cholesterol and triglycerides. "With your family history," Jensen once told me, "it would be my guess that you'd probably develop adult-onset diabetes if you weren't lean, fit and on an excellent diet."

> "A diet rich in w3 fatty acids,... from flax or ... from fish and marine oils, can lower serum triglycerides levels up to 65%. Cholesterol levels may also decrease as much as 25%."

Now, however, it seems I've stumbled onto something to make my diet even better. Both Dr. McDougall and Dr. Simopoulos say that Omega 3 polyunsaturated fats, the kind found in flax seeds and fatty fish, have been shown to lower blood triglyceride levels. What's more, Udo Erasmus, in his encyclopedic *Fats That Heal, Fats That Kill*, says, "A diet rich in w3 fatty acids,... from flax or... from fish and marine oils, can lower serum triglycerides levels up to 65%." Erasmus adds, "Cholesterol levels may also decrease by as much as 25%."

Recall that I added a little over one tablespoon of flax seed oil to my diet before my last visit to the Cooper Clinic, where my triglycerides were found to have dropped below the 100 level for the first time.

In the eight weeks following that exam, I doubled my flax seed intake and added sardines or salmon (both fatty fish) to my evening meal several times a week. My triglycerides then dropped another 20%, to 76. Plus, after an additional two months on this diet, my cholesterol dropped again, to 181.

I believe I'm onto something good. I've made an excellent diet even better—by simply adding a little "good fat."

Don't misunderstand, however. This is not to be interpreted as a license to add fat helter-skelter. My total fat intake is still a low 18%, and the saturated fat in my diet remains a very low 3%. It would not be a advisable to add "good fat" to a diet already high in fat and calories. Adding good fat undoubtedly works best when it replaces saturated fat or refined carbohydrates. Something else seems to be happening. Even though I added about 200 calories of "good fat" to my daily diet, my body weight has not changed. My body fat may even be trending down.

The Saturday morning after I got home from Dallas, the Tanita Body Fat Monitor/Scale registered my fat level at 6%. In the next nine weeks, my Saturday morning readings varied between

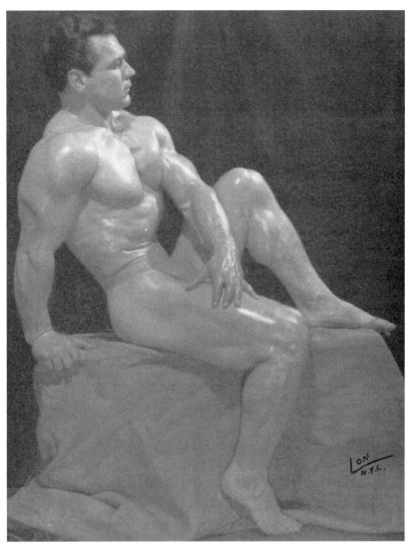

John Grimek once told *Dan Sawyer, who provided this magnificent photo,* that it seemed like everything he did turned to muscle. For a contest, he could put on about 20 pounds of solid flesh—without adding any-thing to his midsection. No telling what Grimek could've done had he known about "good fat."

6.5% and 5.5%, and were as low as 4.5% in the evening when I'm fully hydrated.

This is not supposed to happen—calories do count—but there is at least one mouse study, published in *Metabolism*, that could explain it.

> **The difference in weight between the mice fed a soybean-oil diet and those fed a fish-oil diet is comparable to the difference in weight between a 225- and a 150-pound man.**

In this study, mice prone to diabetes and obesity were raised on a variety of high-fat (60%) diets, all containing the same number of calories. Interestingly, body weight gains varied widely depending on the type of fat consumed. For example, mice fed soybean oil (high in Omega 6 fat) or lard (high in saturated fat) gained far more than those fed fish oil (high in Omega 3).

The discrepancies were startling. According to Dr. Simopoulos, the difference in weight between the mice fed a soybean-oil diet and those fed a fish-oil diet is comparable to the difference in weight between a 225- and a 150-pound man. The lard-fish oil comparison produced a lesser, but still impressive weight gain disparity. Remember, all three diets contained the same number of calories and percentage of fat.

The researchers warn that humans may respond differently, but there sure seems to be something special in fish oil.

One more thing. This study also found some magic in a high-carb diet. Mice fed 63-percent carbohydrates and only 11% fat were just as lean as those fed the fish-oil diet.

Hmmm. Sounds like a low-fat, high-carb diet with a little fish oil added to keep triglycerides in check might be the perfect combination for leanness and health. Remember, however, don't add good fat to a bad diet.

* * * *

Let's turn from the physical to the psychological, and consider the all-important matter of state of mind. Meet a man with a remarkably healthy approach to life.

The Ultimate Challenge

John North is the most positive septuagenarian I know.

In his insightful book *Dare To Be 100*, Walter M. Bortz, M.D., says to determine how old you really are answer the question, "Are you a go-go, slow-go, or no-go?" At the age of 59, facing retirement as a factory worker at General Motors, John North's answer was a resounding "GO."

Dr. Bortz, one of America's most respected and acclaimed authorities on longevity and aging, prescribes a four-pronged plan for living a long, healthy and fulfilling life: Diet, Attitude, Renewal and Exercise (DARE). John North has probably never heard of Bortz, but he is a sterling example of the DARE formula in action.

182

John has always been active both on and off the job, but in his mid-50's he began to experience a sense of physical decline. He began to experience pain in his joints and felt tired a lot. At a height of 5'11" his weight was a stable 170, but he found himself complaining to his wife, "My pants must've shrunk in the wash."

The turning point came in 1982, "when I got super-irritated with myself for being tired during some very heavy digging and cement work when I was doubling the size of my [work] shop." (I told you John has always been active.) Never one to ignore a call to action, he began a program of push-ups that very day. The push-ups worked. They made him stronger and, more importantly, they sent him off in search of a more systematic and complete fitness program.

He found what he was looking for in 1985 while on vacation with his wife. Browsing in a shopping mall bookstore he came upon Arnold Schwarzenegger's *The Education Of A Bodybuilder*. Inspired by what he saw and read in Arnold's book—"I discovered that I didn't have to accept the usual relentless physical decline"—he began to explore the bodybuilding lifestyle. He sent for Arnold's *Basic Guide to Muscle Building and Physical Fitness* and subscribed to *Muscle & Fitness* magazine, where he immediately became interested in my "Ripped Department" and later my books. "For me," John says, "being ripped, especially having a lean and hard abdomen, is the very hallmark of physical fitness." Reflecting further, North added, "My midsection was soft and jiggled a little; I hated that!"

Before long, John had altered his diet. "With my wife's cooperation, I stopped eating the fatty, greasy, oily foods I loved and began eating lots of fresh vegetables, fruits and grains." After getting clearance from his physician he also began a regular, but conservative—"I was cautious about overdoing anything"—program of weight training and fast walking.

It worked beautifully. John's weight soon stabilized at 150, where it has remained for more than a decade. (Check out John's waistline in the following photo.) What's more, the pain in his right shoulder and left knee disappeared, and the world-famous Cleveland Clinic, after a thorough examination, pronounced his heart and circulatory capacity that of a 27-year-old and his blood pressure as youthful as a teenager.

> **"Believe that life is worth living, and your belief will help create the fact."**

That's the D (Diet) and E (Exercise) in Dr. Bortz's DARE prescription. But if that was the whole story, I probably wouldn't

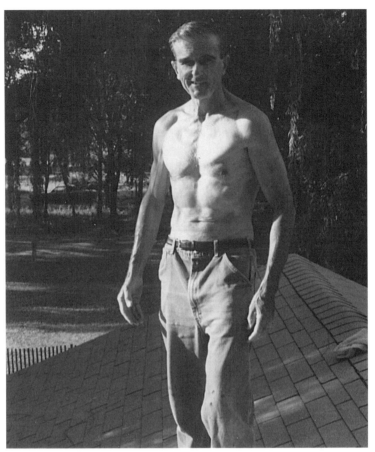

John North in 1987, at the age of 61—looking good, on the roof of his enlarged workshop. *Photo courtesy of John North.*

be telling you about John North. No, where John really shines, what makes him such a standout, is his remarkably positive attitude and his undeniable spirit of renewal, the other two legs of the DARE formula.

Dr. Bortz offers 99 steps that can make the difference between living the usual 75 years or an ideal and successful 100. The most important step, says Bortz, is to believe. "To make 100, you must first believe," he maintains. For Bortz, the belief in 100 means taking up the ultimate challenge to make the most of your life. He quotes from William James' *Will to Believe*: "Believe that life is worth living, and your belief will help create the fact." John North believes.

He just laughs when asked if he isn't too old for bodybuilding. "I accept my age as a natural part of the cycle of life," he says, "but I believe I can maintain my health far above the average for my age." North says, "the greatest gift" of bodybuilding is the attitude: "I can do, I can be, I am a winner, not against others, but for myself." He continues: "The future to me is not a winding-down, but the best of what's to be—the fulfillment of my life's goals, the rewards of a lifetime of effort. The joy of a grandson....There are mountain peaks I want to climb, and I do want to learn to scubadive." You get the idea. John North loves living.

And as if that isn't enough to make Dr. Bortz proud, North also has an unmistakable thirst for renewal. After five years of retirement—he pursued his lifelong hobbies of painting, photography, collecting (stamps, arrowheads, rocks, Civil War items and more) and wrote his autobiography—he went back to work.

John's first post-retirement job was at a greenhouse, where he delighted in keeping up with young workers for eight hours, five days a week. When the greenhouse closed and he was laid off from that job, he became a star employee for a temporary help agency. Most recently, John has been permanently hired by the Superior Roll Forming Company, where he began as a temporary employee.

> "Anyone at any age can be ordinary or average; for myself, I want to work like Michael Jordan plays basketball—I want to be a superstar!"

To give you an idea how pleased John was to achieve permanent full-time status—and how seriously he takes his job— here is a portion of the written statement he presented to the personnel manager:

> My ultimate goals is to personally demonstrate that an 'old' man can also be a high performance worker. I intend to vigorously expand the parameters of what is considered 'able-bodied' among the 'aged.'
>
> I would be profoundly honored if someday someone in Washington recognized what I've tried to do in the workplace after my 'retirement' from General Motors, and thus discover for others the joy I found in being active in my later years. I admit, I don't even think of myself as being old—unless I look in the mirror—but then, a lot depends upon the attitude you have at any age.
>
> Again, thank you for letting me be a member of the Superior Family.

In a letter telling me of his promotion to permanent status, John concluded with a statement I know Dr. Bortz would applaud: "Anyone at any age can be ordinary or average; for myself, I want to work like Michael Jordan plays basketball—I want to be a superstar!"

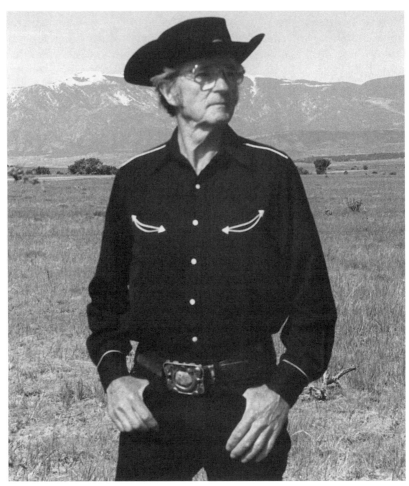

John North today, on the 40-acre spread he recently purchased in Colo-
rado. As optimistic as always, John says, "I feel that this has the potential of becoming the most wonderfully happy time of my life!" By the
way, he can still do 50 push-ups. *Photo courtesy of John North.*

You are, John, you are.

*　*　*　*

Finally, to illustrate the power of self-help and maintaining a
healthy lifestyle, I want to tell you about my latest health and
fitness exam.

Cooper Clinic Fourth Visit—at 60

Results in Brief

Treadmill:	99th percentile
Body fat:	99th percentile

Blood pressure:	105/70
Blood lipids:	"Excellent"
Coronary arteries:	"Very large"
Bone Density:	"Wonderful"
Nutritional Evaluation:	"Just Outstanding"
Exercise Program:	"Well Balanced", "Sensible"

Aerobic Fitness

In reporting on my first visit to the world-famous Cooper Clinic (I was 50), *Muscle & Fitness* contributor David Prokop described the treadmill stress test as a "journey to nowhere." That's because the final destination isn't a place, but a state of total fatigue. The treadmill begins at 3.30 mph on flat and rises 1% each minute (the first grade increase is 2%) up to 25% grade, where the speed increases 0.2 mph for each additional minute. The treadmill always wins, of course; the test is over when the subject can no longer maintain the pace. As you can imagine, it gets quite uncomfortable in the last few minutes as exhaustion approaches. The truth is, for anyone planning to exert a maximum effort it's a little scary. It's a test of will as well as stamina.

My first treadmill test, where I lasted 28 minutes and scored well above the 99th percentile for men 50-59, was the easiest from a mental standpoint. I had no basis for comparison and didn't know what to expect. I just stepped on the moving tread and kept going as long as I could. The next year, when I did even better (29 minutes), was a lot more anxiety producing. Knowing only too well what to expect, I tossed and turned the nights before, agonizing over those last few minutes when anyone in their right mind would want to throw in the towel.

On my last visit, five years ago, I did 28:37. I put too much pressure on myself, however. I overtrained and ended up getting sick on my return home.

This time around my goal was to equal the 28-minute time I did at 50; that was a realistic target. My bodybuilding results convinced me that being 60 was not a limiting factor. About two months out from the test, however, I realized to make 28 minutes I'd have to add more aerobic training. Unfortunately, that would probably cost me some muscle mass and mean less impressive physique photos to mark the end of my sixth decade. (It might also lead to overtraining and illness as it had in 1992.) The choice was between a great treadmill time or great bodybuilding con-

My time was 25 minutes and 15 seconds, which again put me in the 99th percentile for my age group—and in the excellent (87th percentile) category for men in their 30s.

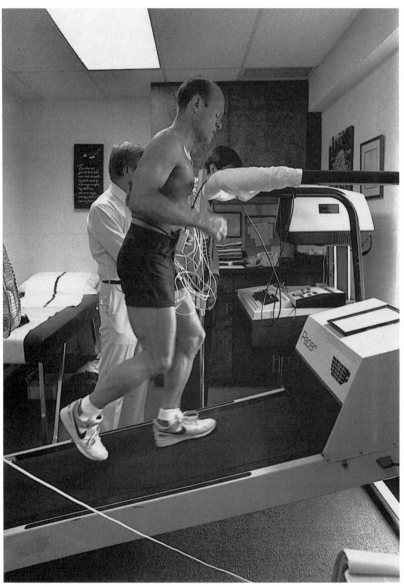

The treadmill is a test of will as well as stamina. *Photo by Justin Joseph.*

dition. I chose the latter. I stuck with my very intense 30-minute aerobic sessions performed once a week (plus walking). It was the correct decision. My photos turned out to be perhaps my best ever. What's more, I slept soundly the night before the test.

My time was 25 minutes and 15 seconds, which again put me in the 99th percentile for my age group—and in the excellent (87th percentile) category for men in their 30s.

Coronary Artery Size and Bone Density

Since my last visit, the Cooper Clinic has installed a new CT scan machine (high-resolution, volume-mode, axial Electron Beam Tomography). In simple terms, the machine allows the doctors to scan your internal organs and bones in tiny slices and visualize the results in 3D on a computer monitor. It's like a tiny space ship moving around inside your body and taking pictures of everything. Dr. Thomas E. Kimball used computer reconstruction to show me the results. Two findings stood out.

First, my coronary arteries are very large, "huge" was the word Dr. Jensen used. Arnie, as Dr. Jensen prefers to be called, says my years of aerobic exercise probably produced the large arteries, which substantially lower my risk of developing obstructive coronary artery disease.

The CT scan also revealed that I have exceptionally good bone mineral content, more than two standard deviations above the norm for my age. As a matter fact, my bone density is more than one standard deviation above the norm for a 20-year-old man. Arnie termed my bone density "wonderful" and attributed it to my long history of weight training.

Nutritional Evaluation

Dr. Jensen had me prepare a daily food record for computer analysis by one of the clinic's registered dieticians. That was easy because I've kept a training diary for years (decades actually) which includes what I eat every day. It's basically the same as the meals described in this book: lots of whole grains, fruits and vegetables, with protein provided by ample quantities of skimmed milk and nonfat plain yogurt, plus a few ounces of chicken or extra-lean beef, and some fatty fish, seeds and nuts to provide essential fat. I also supplement with a few tablespoons of our own milk and egg protein powder and a balanced multi-vitamin/mineral packet. (The protein powder was included in the analysis, but the multi was not.)

I don't calculate the percentage of carbohydrate, protein and fat—I know generally that my diet is high carb, medium protein and low fat—so it was interesting to learn the exact breakdown: complex carbs 58%, protein 29%, fat 12% (saturated 3%, polyunsaturated 4%, monounsaturated 5%) and sugar 1%. (An analysis about six weeks later, after I added a few more seeds and nuts, produced these slightly different results: carbs 56%, protein 26%, and fat 18%)

As explained earlier, I don't count calories. I find it much simpler to follow a uniform eating pattern and monitor my body

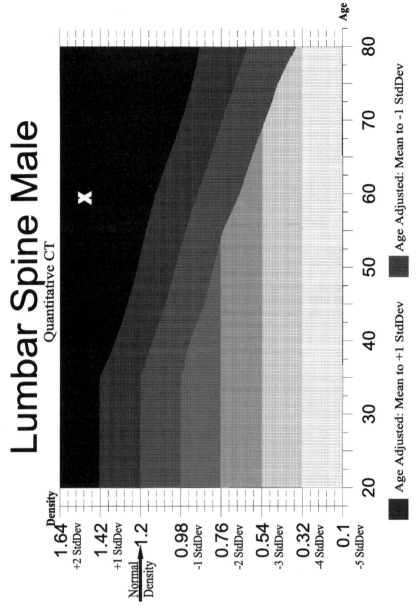

This chart, which is turned sideways, shows my bone density. The "X" indicates that I am considerably *above* the norm for a 20-year-old man. *Chart courtesy of the Cooper Clinic.*

weight and composition. The computer totaled my calorie intake at 2412 (2610 on the subsequent analysis). My dietary fiber as expected, was high at 58 grams. All of my vitamin and mineral requirements were well satisfied (again, without counting the multi).

In his final report, Dr. Jensen wrote, "Your nutritional evaluation is just outstanding....I am very impressed with your diet—good job."

Commenting on my calorie intake, Dr. Jensen observed that the normal intake for a sedentary man my size would be about 1,650, but 2400 is "just about right considering your exercise." My high percentage of active lean tissue, of course, gives me a faster metabolism. My body burns more calories around the clock.

> Dr. Jensen observed that the normal intake for a sedentary man my size would be about 1,650, but 2400 is "just about right considering your exercise."

My protein intake at 29% (179 grams) is higher than the 10-20% usually recommended by dieticians. But it's not high for me, according to Dr. Jensen. "I would recommend that you continue a high protein diet like that," he wrote.

As explained earlier, the latest research shows that hard-training athletes may actually need twice as much protein as an inactive person. Those who work hard at both strength and endurance training (as I do), have the highest protein needs of all athletes.

Still, as my latest evaluation demonstrates, even a person like me, who eats a near-vegetarian diet, can easily meet the newly discovered protein requirements for the hardest training athletes. From the time I took up weight training as a teenager, I've taken care to include some high-quality protein (mostly nonfat dairy products in recent years) with every meal. In the last few decades, however, I've been especially mindful of the fact that excess calories from any source—carbs, fat or protein—build fat, not muscle. Most athletes, especially bodybuilders, grossly overdose on protein.

Words to Live By

Dr. Jensen, a warm and wonderful guy who practices what he preaches—on several occasions Arnie has held the Cooper Clinic treadmill record for his age group—wrapped up his nine page report with these encouraging comments, encouraging not only to me but to anyone trying to live a healthy lifestyle:

> Clarence, I am so impressed by you. You certainly have proven that you can have outstanding strength fitness and aerobic fitness, outstanding percent body fat, excellent lipids, and wonderful bone densities with

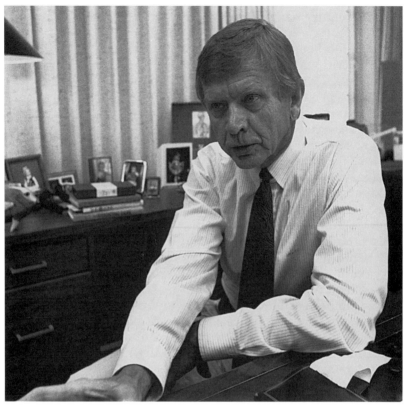

Dr. Arno "Arnie" Jensen (shown here): "The pain of discipline weighs ounces, but the pain of neglect weighs tons." *Photo by Justin Joseph.*

a well-balanced and sensible exercise and dietary program. I think you and I have both proven that consistency and reasonable discipline is the key. The pain of discipline weighs ounces, but the pain of neglect weighs tons. I wish everyone could be half as disciplined and half as consistent as you have been all of your life... If you have got your health and nothing else, you are certainly very rich. If you have all of the material things you want and not your health, I feel you are very poor.

Thanks Arnie—and Amen!

"To be happy, grow."
—George Sheehan, *Personal Best*

CHAPTER SEVEN

People Who Love A Challenge

Five Fascinating People

It seems only logical and right to conclude a book devoted to self challenge with case histories, wonderful examples of the rewards of always trying to improve in some way. The five men profiled here have fascinating and inspiring stories, all quite different. Each has taken a separate and distinct path based on his individual circumstances, strengths, weaknesses and inclinations. Each found something that challenged and excited him, and then pursued it vigorously and consistently.

These are people you'll enjoy reading about, each worthy of a separate biography, but they are also people from whom you can learn. Each has pursued fitness with passion and enthusiasm for decades, most for a lifetime. But they each did it their way, and so should you. They are to be studied and enjoyed, but not necessarily copied or emulated.

Remember the maxim, "Surely the quickest path to disillusionment is the one blazed by someone else." We all have different needs and abilities. Focus on the techniques these men used to pursue their dreams and goals. Take those you can use, apply them to your life, and leave the rest.

One common thread binds all five of these men, however. It's a trait we can all use to enrich our lives. They all set goals for themselves, tasks that taxed but did not overcome their capabilities. They challenged themselves.

Bionic Bill

"Challenge and adversity are often the cornerstone of success," says Bill Clark, a major league baseball scout and a 1997 recipient of the Association of Oldetime Barbell and Strongmen's Highest Achievement Award.

He ought to know. Bill, 66 and the father of five adult children, has turned the challenge of adversity into success in such diverse areas as music, baseball and weightlifting.

At age 10, he learned from countless hours of practice that he had little talent for playing the piano. "Defeat at the keyboard only strengthened my respect for those who master what I could not," Clark says. That experience engendered a deep love for music. "My record library reflects my failure in a positive way," Bill relates. "My life is more serene for having accepted the challenge of the piano—and lost!"

Bill was better at baseball than playing the piano, but he wasn't good enough to realize his dream of becoming a "Big Leaguer." Not willing to let lack of ability stand in his way, he said to himself, "Why not become a Major League umpire?" That didn't work either. Says Bill, "A wife and three children need to eat." He still wasn't ready to give up his dream, however.

After umpiring hundreds of amateur games, Clark had an opportunity to become a scout, and he accepted the challenge. Says Bill, "It meant working in relative obscurity, driving a million miles in 20 years, pushing the body to its limits, but I was a Major Leaguer—Finally!"

As so often happens, that effort opened another door. In 1991, the Atlanta Braves offered Bill the position of international scouting director. I'll let him tell what happened.

> The international game was becoming the new frontier and the Braves offered a huge challenge: Start from scratch and take them to a leadership role. For a guy from the Missouri Ozarks who wore shoes only in winter till he was 12 years old, that's quite a challenge! When you speak English fair and nothing else, that's another challenge. So I hesitated 30 seconds and accepted those challenges. Today, the Braves have had players from 15 different nations on their roster. Atlanta has a physical presence in 50 countries and has taken its place among the elite in international baseball. The challenges, once again, were the cornerstone of success.

Believe it or not, Bill Clark's greatest adversity and challenge have come from weightlifting—with a cruel assist from baseball.

Bill's involvement with the weight sports spans four decades. He was the driving force behind masters (over 40) lifting competition (Olympic and power) both nationally and internationally. In addition, he organized and coordinated prison postal meets for 20 years, and formed the International All-Round Weightlifting Association (IAWA), an organization devoted to all the various odd lifts. In addition to the award mentioned earlier, he's been inducted into seven halls of fame, five lifting, one bowling and one for baseball scouts.

Along the way Bill became a champion performer in the odd lifts that he clearly loves. Again, we'll let him recount his latest run-in with adversity.

> The IAWA helps meet the challenge of aging because it gives a person with less flexibility a chance to lift heavy in such old-time standards as the Hip, Back, Harness and Hand-and-Thigh, among 150 other lifts. After 20 years behind home plate and 38 years as a basketball official, I was faced with joint replacements. Through wear and tear and genetics, I had bone-on-bone in both knees and my hip by 1993. My lifting was minimal. I no longer could run or officiate, walking was a major chore. I was a product of my years. Now came the greatest challenge of my life.

On January 20, 1994, Bill had a rare right knee and right hip replacement. "It was the first time in 14 years the nurses in my ward had seen a knee/hip combo," Bill noted. Ten days later he was able to walk across the room unaided, no cane or crutches. A personally devised pre-operative rehabilitation program made this possible. "I did a lot of heavy Leg Extensions, Leg Presses and Hip Sleds before the surgery and it paid off," he observed. But that was only the beginning.

A return to heavy lifting was out of the question, doctors warned. To which Bill responded, "Hogwash."

A return to heavy lifting was out of the question, doctors warned. To which Bill responded, "Hogwash." Still, he admits to being apprehensive. "Each time I grabbed the iron, I was never sure something wouldn't snap. The first Deadlift at 135 was a thrill—but nothing happened. The first Harness Lift at 875 was scary—but nothing happened."

Don't misunderstand. Bill is no fool. He proceeded with caution. "If there was some discomfort in the hip or knee, I quit," he says. "I never forced the issue." (No one should try this without careful consultation with their doctor.)

In a few months he was deadlifting 450 and the first week in November, 1994, saw him do a 1,435 pound Hip Lift, his best in three years. "The replacements were amazing," Bill reports. "It reduced my strength very little and took away the pain which had dogged me for years." Someone said to the doctor that he had created a monster. "I didn't create one, I just prolonged one," the doctor replied with obvious satisfaction.

Unfortunately, the rare right-side double replacement couldn't

196

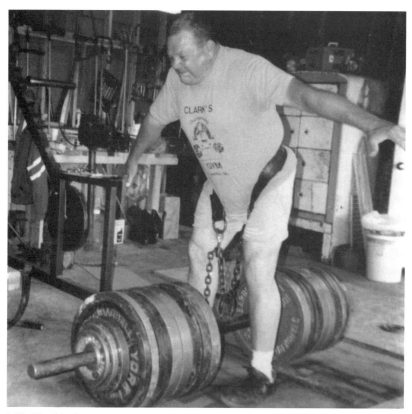

Bill Clark's favorite photo. It shows him doing a Hip Lift of 1,535 pounds—with two new knees and one hip replaced. On the same day, he hoisted 1,620.

cure his other knee, which was also bad. So on November 14, 1994, Bill returned to the hospital for a second knee replacement. "I might not be able to lift again," he said before the surgery.

As you probably guessed, Bill beat the odds again. Ten and one-half weeks after the second knee replacement, he did a 460 Deadlift in competition and had 500 half way up. "That was my best in three years," he said. "I hadn't done 500 in six years." His poundages astonished everyone, especially the doctors— "mainly because no one has tried them before," Bill explains, downplaying his remarkable achievement.

"Why did you do it, Bill?" I asked. "I like a challenge," he replied. "I can't imagine just sitting down after replacement surgery; it's not my style. I'm amazed how people give in to something as uncomplicated as rehabing a replacement."

At this point, however, the story takes another turn for the worse. Listen to Bill again.

I had set three goals. I challenged myself to walk 100 miles in 24 hours, to deadlift 500 and to harness lift 1000 kilos [2206 lbs]. For a 65-year-old, these are attainable goals; for a 65-year-old with three new joints, this was uncharted territory.

The 500 Deadlift became possible when I did 480 and the 1000-kg was beaten in a gym workout. To do it officially, I took 2,215 lbs. in a sanctioned record day. My left hip had been a problem and on this day, when the weight cleared the floor the left hip gave to the right and the 1000 kilos shifted over the right leg, snapping the right tibia like a match stick. So much for 1000 kilos.

Now, the real dues of challenge began.

After spending seven months with his right leg in a cast, Bill's remaining natural hip, the left, had to be replaced. Like before, he was back to a 440 Deadlift only two months after the replacement. "At least the 500 Deadlift and the century walk seemed within reach," Bill says now. "I knew the 1000-kg Harness might have to wait."

Rather than improvement, however, the next 18 months brought more adversity. Bill's left hip dislocated four times and had to be replaced again. During the repair, the femoral nerve was bruised, leaving most of the muscles of Bill's left leg without stimulation. "From January, 1997, to August, 1998, I had not a single workout," he says.

Nevertheless, he refused to be grounded during the months of inactivity. He continued his globe-trotting ways, with an essentially lifeless left leg, traveling 400,000 miles in pursuit of talent for the Braves. Talk about meeting a challenge head-on!

That's where Clark's "saga of the joints" stands as of this writing. Was it worth it, Bill? Any second thoughts?

Adversity made it very difficult during the past five years to meet the challenges I imposed on myself, but they are no different than getting to the Major Leagues, or learning to play the piano.

If I fail to deadlift 500 pounds, become a Centurian, or make 1000 kilos in the Harness, I can relax with a piano concerto which I could never play and live with the knowledge that at least the challenge was met, if not overcome.

I can't imagine not having tried.

Best of luck, Bill. You are a living testament that God helps those who help themselves.

Hilligenn Does It Better

Always ready for a challenge, Roy Hilligenn, the 1951 Mr. America, used to boast, "I can do anything you can do—and better." And more often than not it was true! John Grimek said Hilligenn had the "biggest mouth in the business," but he "could back it up."

Believe it or not, nothing has changed. At 76, Roy can still "do it better."

Not long ago, *The Iron Master* (199 S.E. 10th Court, Hermiston, Oregon 97838, 1-541-667-8123), edited by Osmo "John" Kiiha, did a wide-ranging interview with Hilligenn. After talking to Roy over several months, covering everything from childhood to the present day, Kiiha wrote, "Hilligenn is one of the best advertisements for modern bodybuilding." Roy is living proof of the fruits of eating well and training hard for a lifetime. "Over a half century into the [iron] game, Roy is still…very much the strong man of his earlier years," Kiiha said. As you'll see, when it comes to physical strength and stamina, Hilligenn has given new meaning to the word longevity.

> **When it comes to physical strength and stamina, Hilligenn has given new meaning to the word longevity.**

Roy began weight training in South Africa, where he was born in 1922. His father died when he was four. Unable to cope with the situation, his mother was forced to place him in an orphanage, where he remained for 11 years. At 15, he began studying to become an electrician. After two years, he began work as an apprentice and soon thereafter had a serious accident. He slipped while connecting a neon sign on the roof of a hotel and fell four stories. He suffered internal injuries and a broken wrist and several fingers.

Hospitalized for nine months, he came out at 18, weighing only 83 pounds (at 5'6") with a hand that wouldn't open. Roy received no physical therapy in the hospital. Left to his own devices, he discovered a crude form of progressive exercise while attempting to restore function to his crippled hand.

The story of the restoration shows Roy's determination. He first tried pounding a punching bag, but that did nothing to open his hand. Roy told Osmo Kiiha what he did next:

> I would take a walk to the dumps, looking for something, I don't know what. One day I found a pair of solid steel wheels, weighing 35 pounds. I lifted that thing with my left hand eventually. My right hand was crippled and couldn't grip it, it wouldn't open. So I

squeezed a piece of wire through my fist—the blood came out the opposite side. I tied that to a bucket of water, trying to force the hand open. Eventually I could squeeze a little rubber tube in there, and I would squeeze and squeeze, then the inside rubber ball from a golf ball, then a bigger ball, then a pair of socks, and a tennis ball. Then I could grip the steel wheels. It got better and better.

With that success under his belt, Roy was ready for new challenges. Like many others of the time, he was inspired to take up weight training after seeing a photo of John Grimek on the cover of *Strength & Health*. Working out with a set of homemade weights given to him by a neighbor, Roy's weight went from 83 to 101 in the first year. In spite of the meager gains, he kept on pumping. In the next six months, his weight jumped to 148, and then to 159 by the end of the year. The second year gains were a portent of what was to come.

He did 180 in the Press and Snatch and 240 in the Clean & Jerk, even though he'd never seen anybody do the lifts before.

Roy's first contest was an accident. His interest peaked by an ad in the newspaper, he arrived early at the venue of a novice lifting event, and was standing at the front of the line waiting to get in when the promoter spotted him. "You going to enter?" he asked. "Oh no, I know nothing about contests, I just come to see," Roy replied. "I can see you work out," the man said. Roy had never lifted more than the 145 pounds he had at home. "I can lift that 10 times," he told the man.

The promoter took him backstage and showed him the trophies and the first Olympic lifting set he'd ever seen. "I bent over, spun the bar, I was so excited I nearly kissed that bar and weights," Roy told Osmo. The man said, "Look, you can take a trophy home tonight." That did it.

Roy entered and won! He did 180 in the Press and Snatch and 240 in the Clean & Jerk, even though he'd never seen anybody do the lifts before. Roy also placed 2nd in the physique contest held along with the lifting.

The rest, as they say, is history. Says Roy, "I set my goals, and achieved more than I bargained for." He won the Mr. South Africa title in 1943, 1944, 1946 and 1975. He was also the first South African to Clean & Jerk double bodyweight. His lifts in 1946 were 245 Press, 255 Snatch and 321 Clean & Jerk. As mentioned earlier, he eventually won the 1951 Mr. America,

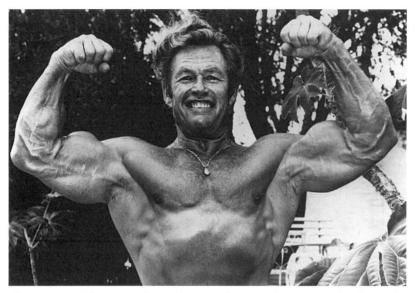

This is Roy in his 50s, at about the time he won the Mr. South Africa title for the fourth time. He was truly a smiling superman. *Photo courtesy of the Todd-McLean Collection.*

which at that time was the most prestigious physique title in the world.

Had he not injured himself prior to the event, Roy probably would have also won the U.S. National Weightlifting Championship, which was held along with the Mr. America contest.

Shortly before the contest, Roy did a Dead Hang Clean with 375 for 5 reps and one jerk. "I was ready and convinced of setting world records with at least 935 or better total," says Roy. But lightning struck only three days out from the contest. "I was only using 280 pounds for Speed Cleans and did a set of 12 reps," he told Kiiha. "I pulled the weight on the last rep so hard it threw me flat on my butt, the weight going over my head. I hung on to the bar and somehow sprained both my wrists. I was in agony. On the day of the contest I could barely lift a glass of water." Nevertheless, with his wrists tightly bandaged, Roy managed to do 240-260-330 to place second to the world's best 198 pounder, Norbert Schemansky, who totalled 915.

The next year, Roy won the Junior National Championship as a 181 pounder. (The Junior Nationals were open to anyone who had not won that meet or the Senior Nationals.) His lifts were 260-245-

At a later date, he did a 375 Clean & Jerk at a bodyweight of 173, equal to the then-world record.

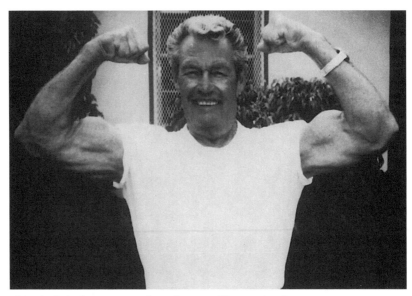

This slightly fuzzy snapshot shows Hilligenn in the same pose—at 75. Roy says his biceps are 18" cold. *Photo courtesy of Roy Hilligenn.*

335. On an extra attempt he Cleaned and Jerked 350, which was eight pounds more than double bodyweight.

At a later date, he did a 375 Clean & Jerk at a bodyweight of 173, equal to the then-world record. What's more, as if his lifting wasn't enough to demonstrate his athletic ability, Roy would often entertain the crowd by doing a series of back flips across the stage.

Interestingly, Roy is a vegetarian. "I was born a vegetarian, I think," he told Osmo Kiiha. "Since infancy I never liked meat, never ate it, never ate turkey, chicken, fish or eggs. I am still a vegetarian." Most of his protein came from milk and soy. "I always drank about a gallon [of milk] a day, I still do," he said.

Says Roy, "I'm so healthy it's embarrassing. If I felt any better I'd have to see a doctor." In addition to exercise, he believes the reason is his diet. "I truly believe that fruit is the body's cleanser, vegetables are the body's healer, and meat is the body's premature aging agent and the cause of all diseases except virus disease."

I said at the outset that Roy can still "do it better." In a letter written in April of 1998, when he was 75 and weighed 160, Roy told me, "I can still Squat 405 lbs., Two Hand Deadlift 520, and One Hand Deadlift 400 lbs. any day." As an aside, he mentioned that in 1978 he made a world record in the One Hand Deadlift with 550 pounds. The record still stands, he said.

In addition, Roy confirmed a mind-boggling feat of strength and endurance reported earlier by Osmo Kiiha. It was performed in March 1995, when he was 72.

> We had a contest for the Deadlift, doing repetitions, no belt, and no straps were allowed. The finalists were a man who weighed 264, one who weighed 235, and [me] at 165. We had to take a 400 lb. barbell, and see how many reps we could do; we could take 2-10 seconds rest to regrip the bar. The first man [235 lbs.] could do only 9 reps, claiming back trouble, the big guy did 29 reps and I did 35 reps!

No doubt about it, Roy. You're The Man.

Beyond Fitness

In 1989, George Sheehan wrote in *Runner's World* about a friend who taught a much-in-demand fitness course at a state university. The protocol was not unusual, weights one day and jogging the next, yet the students rarely dropped out. The reason, Sheehan explained, was because it was a mountain-climbing course. The students were preparing to climb Mt. Hood.

"The mountain transforms this fitness program into a challenging experience," wrote Sheehan. "It changes something boring into something exciting."

Sheehan's point, of course, was that you need a goal to give meaning to your training. Otherwise, as Sheehan put it, you "start to feel like Sisyphus forever pushing the stone, yet never arriving at a goal."

I've used this story many times, in writing and speaking, to illustrate the critical importance of goal-setting, but it was only recently that it dawned on me that Sheehan's friend was one and the same as my friend Dr. Pat O'Shea, Professor Emeritus of exercise and sports science at Oregon State University.

> To use Sheehan's metaphor, there has always been a challenging mountain at the end of Pat's training program.

A modest man, Pat let me figure this out entirely on my own. Even though I sent him a video of a speech I made to a Boy Scout group prominently featuring his course, he didn't say a word. Only after I put two and two together and asked him point blank—twice—did he admit to being a longtime friend of Dr. Sheehan.

It was obvious after I learned more about O'Shea's background. To use Sheehan's metaphor, there has always been a challenging mountain at the end of Pat's training program.

Pat can't recall a time when he wasn't involved in physical activity. His mother was a world-class long distance swimmer in the early 1930s, and fitness was a way of life for the whole family. They hiked, swam and rode bikes. Significantly, Pat says, "We never thought of doing these activities as exercise." For his sports-oriented family, "being physical fit was simply the norm," says O'Shea.

Pat and his wife Susie have raised their three children in the same environment. From their earliest years, the O'Shea children experienced fitness as "just part of life," says Pat. No baby sitters for them, the O'Shea kids did all the outdoor activities—backpacking, snow camping, cross-country skiing—in which their parents were involved. "At the time," says Pat, "I don't think they really understood the significance of their outdoor lifestyle which taught them to be self-sufficient and rely on themselves while still looking out for others." Living in Oregon and doing all the physically challenging outdoor activities, the whole family had to be in a constant state of what Pat calls "ready fitness." "Due to the risks and dangers involved, you can't afford not to be [fit]," says Pat. "To this day, for me and my family [being physically fit] is the accepted life style."

Weightlifting entered Pat's life after he graduated from high school, where he had been on the swim team. "I continued to

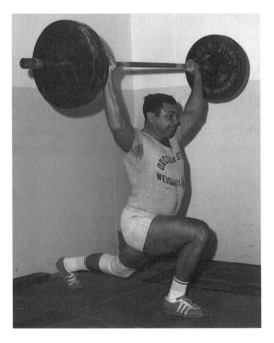

Pat was a competitive Olympic lifter for 13 years. This photo, taken in 1965, shows him doing a heavy Snatch in the split style. *Photo courtesy of Pat O'Shea.*

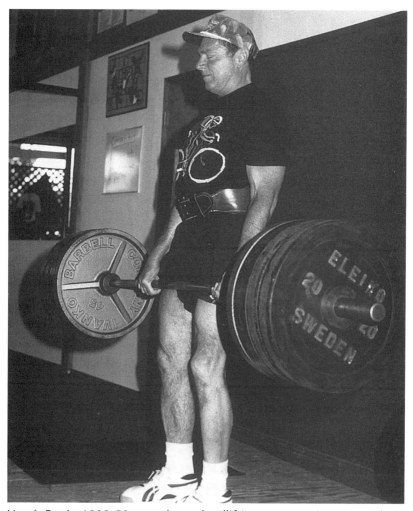

Here's Pat in 1998, 33 years later, deadlifting some serious iron. *Photo courtesy of Pat O'Shea.*

swim at the local YMCA, where in order to enter the pool you had to pass through the weightlifting area which was quite fascinating to me," says Pat. "Eventually I began spending more time with the weights than swimming."

After receiving some coaching from one of the lifters at the Y, a former heavyweight junior national champion by the name of Al Kornke, Pat went on to become an outstanding Olympic lifter—at a bodyweight of 181, he did a 270 Standing Press, 276 Snatch and 342 Clean & Jerk—and power lifter, where his best lifts were 357 Bench Press, 607 Squat and 629 Deadlift. Many years later, Pat is still lifting heavy weights. He recently celebrated his 67th birthday by making the following lifts at a bodyweight of 188: Squat 375, Power Clean 220, Deadlift 450 and Bench Press 225. (The Squat was a conservative effort because he'd strained a knee a few weeks before.)

Pat is more than a strength athlete, of course. His talents extend beyond lifting to endurance sports. He's an accomplished cyclist, mountain climber, skier and coach. For the last 15 years, he has competed in senior masters competition in cycling, triathlons and powerlifting.

Interestingly, Pat's training rotates with the seasons. From November to March, he focuses on powerlifting, stationary biking and cross-country skiing. The rest of the year, April to October, he does cycling, backpacking and other mountaineering activities. Clearly, he's never bored.

Pat is truly a Renaissance man. He's done it all. But, his new book, Quantum Strength, published in 1996, may be his crowning achievement.

In the academic realm, Pat has been a student of sports physiology for more than four decades. His textbook, *Scientific Principles and Methods of Strength Fitness*, published in 1976, sold over 75,000 copies and was considered the bible of strength training. He has authored over 125 articles which have been published in both professional journals and mass media publications. He's widely sought as a lecturer and for clinics in cycling, track & field, skiing, triathlons and mountaineering.

Pat is truly a Renaissance man. He's done it all. But, his new book, *Quantum Strength*, published in 1996, may be his crowning achievement.

Pat says he's been preparing to write this book for 30 years. It represents the culmination of his experiences as a competitive Olympic lifter (13 years), strength coach (Oregon State University 1965-76), professor of exercise and sports physiology (29 years), and multi-sport athlete. "In writing this book, I have integrated scientific principles and concepts of gender-free athletic-type strength training together with applied methods of multi-sport cross-training which will provide an athlete with the knowledge necessary to achieve his or her potential."

Now that you know Pat O'Shea's background, you can understand why students lined up to take his mountaineering course. He walks his talk. Obviously, he knows how to make fitness challenging and fun.

I asked Pat to sum up his philosophy of fitness. Here's his thoughtful response:

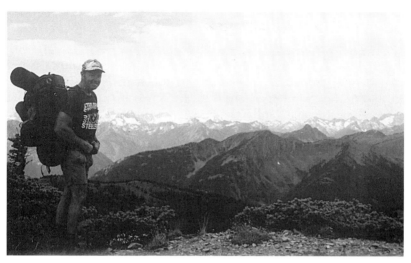

Pat in mountaineering mode, hiking the rugged Pacific Crest Trail in Washington's North Cascades Wilderness. He and wife Susie, over a five year period, backpacked from the Oregon/California border up to Canada, a distance of 800 miles. *Photo courtesy of Pat O'Shea.*

First off, let me say that I'm not a fitness "geek." I appreciate the "good life" too much—good wine, good food, and beautiful women. My life in general has been a physical adventure with fitness playing a major role in shaping it. And while I don't consider fitness to be the end product of training, it has been the source of my freedom to cycle, run, swim, ski, climb mountains, and play games. The physical demands of these activities have served as a motivating force behind a life-long commitment to fitness.

One of the abstract values of masters competition is that it has enabled me to experience the same emotional and physical highs I felt 30 years ago when executing a heavy Snatch or Clean in competition. Training for masters competition keeps my mind and aging body flexible and in working harmony. With each passing decade of life the desire to physically excel serves as the primary motivating force behind my training. Too, I'm most grateful to our creator for giving me the health and wisdom to pursue a vigorous and challenging life.

Thanks Pat. You're a role model for anyone who wants to challenge himself or herself for a lifetime.

207

Six Decade Pilgrimage

George Sheehan, the very wise philosopher mentioned in connection with Pat O'Shea, said that people won't exercise just because it's good for them. The key to motivating people to train, he contended, is inspiration. Bob Hoffman and Joe Weider must have come to essentially the same conclusion many years ago when they began their respective publishing careers. The bigger-than-life stars of muscledom featured in their magazines from the beginning have inspired countless wide-eyed readers to take up bodybuilding. Some, I suspect, are incredulous at first, because the bodies in the magazines are unlike anything they've seen in person. That was my reaction—until I spotted Jim Schwertley in the locker room of the Albuquerque YMCA.

> **His pecs and abs rippled as he pulled on the shirt—and his arms. Oh, those arms!**

It was about 45 years ago, and I still remember it well. In those days, the YMCA was the local hotbed of lifting. That's where the hard-core weightmen trained. I don't remember why I was there, because I was a rank beginner training at home. What I do remember, however, is seeing Jim Schwertley dressing after a workout. I watched him slip a clean white T-shirt over his head and pull up his suspenders. I didn't get a good look at his torso, just a glimpse really, but it was enough to make a lifelong impression.

His pecs and abs rippled as he pulled on the shirt—and his arms. Oh, those arms! As he adjusted his suspenders, to my young eyes they looked like hams bursting out of his sleeves! That was it. But it was enough to convince me that weight training really could accomplish miracles. It was like seeing Popeye in the flesh. The thought of it still makes me want to train.

Many years later, I received a call from Jim Schwertley. He ordered some of my books and, in passing, mentioned that he served with the Air Force in Albuquerque in the early '50s. He wondered if I might remember him. I think it surprised him when I said, "I sure do." I don't believe we had ever spoken before. I delighted in telling him of my reaction to seeing him in the locker room that day long ago. I also related how impressed I was with his overall physique when I saw him in the Mr. New Mexico contest. I don't recall his placing (I think he came in behind soon-to-be Mr. America Steve Klisanin). But I remembered his massive thighs and especially how he could control his abdominal muscles, relaxing the rectus abdominis on one side while contracting the other, making his abs literally dance

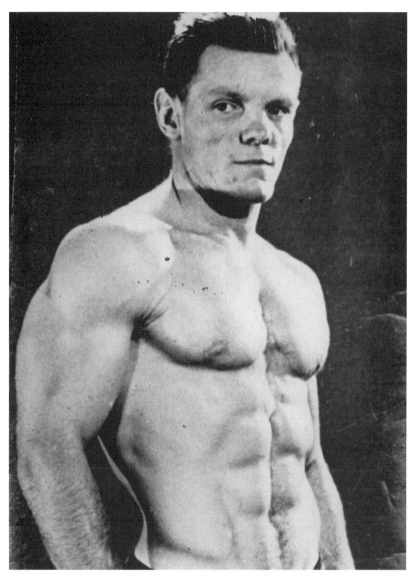

Spotting Jim Schwertley in the locker room of the Albuquerque YMCA was like seeing Popeye in the flesh. As you can see from this photo, taken at the time, he was the genuine article. *Photo courtesy of Jim Schwertley.*

back and forth. He was the whole package, just like the physiques in the magazines.

Jim had previously won the Mr. Omaha (1949) and the Midwest district championship (1951). A year later, in 1952, he won the Nebraska championship in both physique and lifting, and entered the Mr. America contest. He went on to win three state and regional championships in lifting and to qualify for the nationals, before retiring from competition in 1956.

In 1994, Jim passed through Albuquerque on vacation and Carol and I shared a most enjoyable afternoon with him. Among other things, we learned that he entered the seminary soon after being discharged from the Air Force and was ordained as a Catholic priest in 1961. He later sent us an 11-page biography his parishioners put together in 1986 to celebrate the 25th anniversary of his ordination. He's had a wonderfully successful and varied career. His parishioners, who clearly respect and love him, described Father Jim as a "priest, educator, counselor, athlete, philosopher, writer, author, journalist, homilist, retreat director, actor, playwright, scholar, brother, nephew and friend." Among his many accomplishments, Jim is probably best known as a nationally acclaimed lecturer and counselor in the field of alcohol and drug dependency. What's more, he still pumps iron regularly at 70. Obviously, I could not have picked a better source of inspiration.

Jim and I have been in regular contact since his first visit. We've become good friends. One of the things I like best is Jim's sense of humor. He wrote a humor column for the seminary newspaper and later for *The Catholic Voice*. Fond of making fun of himself, he insists that the highlight of his college years at Creighton University was making the "top 20" in the semi-finals of the McShane speech contest. The "triumph" was later diminished, he says, when he failed to make the finals; he forgot all but the first line in his speech and finished last. "It was memorable in a negative way, [because] it was probably the worst speech in the history of the McShane contest, nine words and two gestures," Jim recalls.

> "My desire for strength and fitness started at the age of nine, 61 years ago. I was undersized, young for my school class and had large protruding ears that resembled open Volkswagen doors."

Jim's humor comes through as he recounts his physical culture pilgrimage. Laugh and learn as he tells how he managed to pursue weight training with "unabated enthusiasm" for six decades. Note in particular Jim's effective use of meaningful goals and inspirational role models.

"My desire for strength and fitness started at the age of nine, 61 years ago. I was undersized, young for my school class and had large protruding ears that resembled open Volkswagen doors. This made me an intriguing target for local bullies who

210

seemed to have a vast conspiracy to spook me. Fortunately, my father saw my predicament as I raced home one day, pursued by a gang of tiny toughs. They were under the leadership of a husky kid who, though only in the third grade, had already built a fearsome image in the neighborhood. The fact that he had eyebrows that came together in the middle like kissing caterpillars enhanced his menace. When his gang lurked around the school yard, I was as nervous as a mouse at a cat convention.

"My father gave me my first goal, learn to box, called the 'art of self defense' in those days. I faithfully struggled through lessons at the local Athletic Club. The only other kid in the class, a tall, skinny lad, was convenient to spar with as I learned how to deal with a larger opponent. We were forced to learn the fundamentals by our persuasive coach, especially the left jab. It was like the 'Karate Kid' movie, only with boxing. My father bought me some gloves and often got down on his knees to spar with me. He also got me a heavy punching bag to pummel with my tiny fists. All this strengthened my muscles and confidence, starting a liking for training routines which gave a sense of accomplishment and progress. The bullies backed off when I used my newfound skills to zing a couple of them. Mighty Mouse had struck back. No self respecting bully wanted to take the risk of being zapped by a pygmy with big ears. The lessons I learned in that year engendered a desire for further strength and skill, which I put to work on a swimming team at the club, a kid hockey team and grade school football. My father and the boxing coach had been great role models.

"But I was still a runt, a healthy runt, but a runt—5'1" and 105 pounds at the age of 15. One day, lamenting that I was too small for high school football, I saw an ad depicting Charles Atlas advertising 'Dynamic Tension' which he said had built him up and was the secret of the strength of the tigers in the jungle. Sounded good to me! It also rung a memory bell when he showed the ad depicting the former 97-pound weakling waylaying the bully who had kicked sand in his face the year before. I wasn't interested in getting revenge on any more of the bullies but coveted a build like Atlas. The ad showed him as tanned and majestic with a pearly smile. I ordered the course and worked for a year with some regularity on push-ups, chins, isometrics, and isotonics which were staples of the course. Results were slow. I could do 50 push-ups but had gained only 15 pounds. I did grow four inches, which would have happened anyway. The free-hand training seemed dull and repetitive. Also, I wasn't approaching the Atlas physique. I couldn't even match his sun tan.

"Then another role model appeared in the form of a five foot,

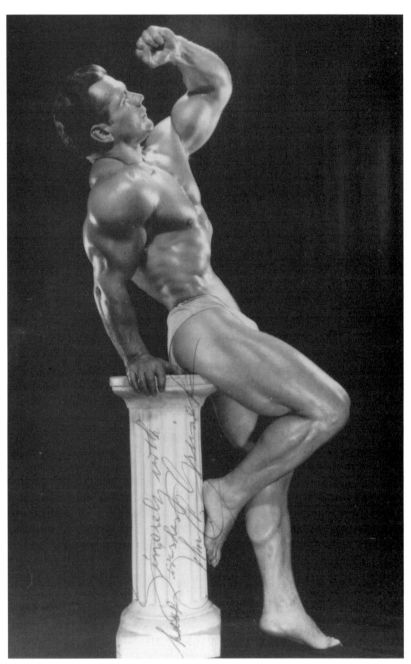

John Grimek's classic pedestal pose inspired Schwertley and many others to embark on a lifetime quest for physical excellence. It may very well be the greatest physique photograph of all time. *Photo courtesy of the Todd-McLean Collection.*

160-pound Navy V-12 cadet in wartime training at a nearby university gym. That little block of granite was striking, my first flesh and blood muscle man sighting. He told me he got that way lifting weights. So, looking past the Superman section at the local drug store, I discovered *Strength & Health* magazine, and the fledgling *Your Physique* published by a young Joe Weider. I ordered the York weights with financial help from my parents and began training on July 6, 1945, at the age of 16, all 5'5" and 120 pounds of zeal and gristle.

> "I decided I would rather be a muscle-bound hulk than a flexible runt, and besides, I could always get a crew cut."

"Two months later, I was still plugging away, focusing on the muscular sailor I had seen the year before. Some people warned me not to use weights or I would get muscle-bound and not be able to comb my hair. I decided I would rather be a muscle-bound hulk than a flexible runt, and besides, I could always get a crew cut. Progress continued to be slow and I began to fear that I might have trouble reaching muscular mediocrity.

"Then it happened. In September, 1945, I spied a *Strength & Health* cover depicting a fabulous specimen, a man named John Grimek perched on a pedestal. I was awestruck by the size, shape, symmetry and chest/waist differential of this otherworldly figure. It jump started my training to a new dimension and it hasn't abated since. It was a key moment of inspiration and I set a goal to get as close to that quality as I could. The picture continues to be an inspiration to this day, like the statue of David by Michelangelo might inspire an artist. I hung it on the wall along with other pictures in a basement gym, the only one in town at the time. I have a framed copy of that classic pedestal pose, which I still consider the greatest physique shot ever taken. I continued to follow the muscle magazines regularly and particularly liked *Iron Man* published by Peary Rader, who I later visited at his home in Alliance, Nebraska.

"Starting training, I had a goal of 150 pounds bodyweight in a year, and a 150 pound Clean & Jerk. Missed the weight by five pounds but exceeded the lift by 20. The second year the goal was 160 pounds and a lift of 200, both reached. The third year it was to win the Mr. Omaha physique title which failed but I made it the next year. I got my first regular training partner at that time, a young man in law school plus many others who came and went. I never missed a workout in ten years. I worked on the Olympic lifts every springtime and set a goal of a 300 pound Clean & Jerk by the age of 25. I made the lift, which was significant since it was the first time 300 had been officially lifted in

Nebraska. I liked the lifting contests better than the physique events, but not many lifters competed. I made a goal to win state and district physique events and regional ones, which I did except I only got to second in the regionals. I did compete in the Mr. America in 1952 while in the Air Force. At 5'8" and 180, I didn't place but took 3rd in the "Best Abdominals" category.

"During the Korean war, I started a bodybuilding program at Kirtland Air Force base in New Mexico and worked out at the Albuquerque YMCA with a large collection of sinewy characters, the best of which was Steve Klisanin, a future Mr. America. After the war I returned to Nebraska and tapered off competitions as I was planning to enter the seminary. I entered in 1956 and took a 1000 pounds of weights along. As I loaded them into the little room below the gym, the monk who ran the seminary was reputed to have inquired: "Has that guy ever done time?" I had quite a few training partners at the seminary, three in par-

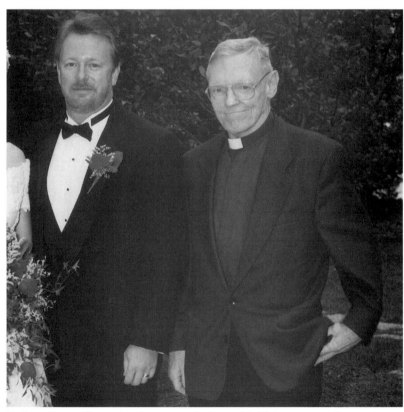

Father Jim still pumps iron regularly at 70. This recent photo shows him "in uniform" after performing a wedding ceremony. *Photo courtesy Father Schwertley.*

ticular who labored at what we called the "sweatshop," part of an old locker room. "After becoming a priest in 1961, I concentrated mostly on working out in gyms which were being opened at that time. I went at least twice a week and trained early in the morning at the rectory once a week. I have had only three regular training partners, for two years apiece, during the 37 years since I left the seminary, but I stayed with it.

"The big factor in staying motivated, in addition to goal setting, always trying to improve in some way, keeping in touch with expert advice and role models, is the sense of well being, energy, health, and strength training gives."

"I contacted John Grimek several times over the years for training advice, and received help and encouragement each time. In the 1980's, I became fond of articles by Clarence Bass in *Muscle & Fitness* magazine. Later I contacted him, bought his books, and visited him several times in Albuquerque.

"The big factor in staying motivated, in addition to goal setting, always trying to improve in some way, keeping in touch with expert advice and role models, is the sense of well being, energy, health, and strength training gives. (I haven't had a cold in 20 years.) Except for going to church, it is the best habit I've ever had."

Thanks for telling us your wonderful story, Jim. I thought you were terrific when my young eyes spotted you in the locker room of the Albuquerque Y, but you're even more inspirational now!

Doctor Heavyhands

In February 1995, my phone rang. The soft-spoken caller said, "You may or may not remember me; this is Len Schwartz." With only a moment's hesitation, I responded, "Sure, I remember you; you're Dr. Schwartz, the Heavyhands man. I first learned about whole-body aerobics from your book."

Leonard Schwartz, M.D., invented Heavyhands. Heavyhands is a system of aerobic exercise using light dumbbells, 1-15 pounds, for high repetitions, up to 30 minutes or more. We've all seen walkers pumping small hand weights. Well, they probably got the idea from reading Dr. Schwartz's *Heavyhands* book, published in 1982. His basic contention is that four limbs are better than two for expending calories and burning fat, that you can continue exercising longer at the same intensity than you can using only the legs.

Schwartz, a psychiatrist, came up with the idea for Heavyhands about five years before the publication of his book, after two years of running and swimming. Prior to that, he says, "I don't think I had ever run 300 yards nonstop before my fiftieth birthday."

After two years of traditional aerobics, at 52, he'd lowered his resting heart rate from 80 to 60 and reduced his body fat from 15 percent to 14 percent. Not bad, but things really took off when he started doing Heavyhands. By the time he was 57, his resting pulse was a phenomenal 38 and his body fat had dropped to 4 percent. His oxygen uptake capacity moved up from what you'd expect for a sedentary physician to a level on par with world-class marathon runners and cross-country skiers. From age 50 to 57, he reduced his bodyweight from a moderately lean 147 to 132 pounds of sinewy muscle. He's not a big man, but his definition and muscularity would make bodybuilders half his age sit up and take notice. Dr. Schwartz says Heavyhands worked some physiological miracles on him, and obviously it did.

When Len Schwartz called me, it was 13 years after the publication of *Heavyhands*. We proceeded to have a nice chat. He was 69, and still going strong. He weighed about the same, 135 pounds, and was working out with Heavyhands every day. Incredibly, he'd recently pumped 6-pound weights at a 110 stride/ stroke-per-minute pace for 200 minutes—in a semi-duckwalk position! Moreover, he had another book out, which he promised to send me.

A few days later an autographed copy of *The Heavyhands Walking Book!* arrived with a letter from Len saying he wanted to sell me "on the notion of gaining strength (admittedly a different species of it!) during aerobic sessions." Needless to say, I was eager to read Schwartz's second offering, which puts forth his ideas on a new form of fitness.

We've all heard claims that hand weights add little to the workload or fitness benefits of walking. Dr. Schwartz says that's true, if you merely carry the weights at your sides. "Even huge weights don't evoke much aerobic work when hanging inertly," he explains. "You have to act boldly," pumping your arms high and fast. "Pumping 3-pound weights 3 feet up and down at 110 beats/minute convert a 2.5-mph walk to the equivalent of a 6-mph jog," Schwartz asserts. In short, pump height, Schwartz calls it "verticality," drives intensity.

Dr. Schwartz stresses verticality in both books. What's new is his contention that Heavyhands training produces a unique form of fitness. He calls this separate fitness factor "strength-endurance fitness," claiming it is more than simply strength plus endurance. "The best proof of that is that the strongest strength

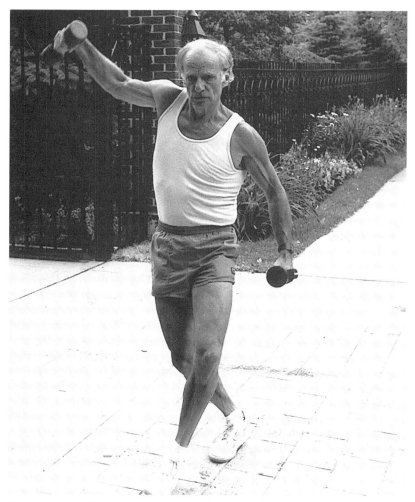

The inventor of Heavyhands, 64 in this photo, shows how it's done. *Photo courtesy Len Schwartz, M.D.*

athletes don't enjoy much of it," he asserts, "and the best pure endurance athletes don't either." Strength-endurance, according to Dr. Schwartz, is gained through strength-endurance training, such as that offered by Heavyhands movements for the whole body.

Pure endurance training, such as running, he points out, does not build strength. On the other hand, he says, strength training in which muscle groups are isolated and exercised in sequence does not produce strength-endurance. According to Dr. Schwartz, strength-endurance is only produced when as much muscle as possible is loaded simultaneously and for a prolonged period of time. Heavyhands strength walking as described in

217

The Heavyhands Walking Book!, says Dr. Schwartz, is an ideal training strategy for those seeking strength-endurance.

There's merit in what Dr. Schwartz says. As noted earlier in this book, it is well known that the results of exercise are quite specific (SAID). It's axiomatic that runners should run, swimmers should swim, rowers should row and lifters should lift. By this line of reasoning, if you want to be able to pump hand weights high and fast, like Dr. Schwartz, then you should train as he suggests. You'll likely end up with a body stronger and more muscular than a runner, but with less strength and muscle mass than a bodybuilder. You'll probably be proportioned like Len Schwartz, with more muscular development in the upper body than the lower. You'll be very lean (if you watch your diet), and your whole body will be aerobically fit. As Dr. Schwartz points out—quite correctly, I believe—many prefer this type of body.

> **Confronted with the need to counter a rapidly aging body, most people would follow the herd and do what everybody does (jog, bike, swim, lift weights), but not Len Schwartz.**

Four years have passed since Len rang me up the first time, and we've become friends by phone, letter and e-mail. My Dad, a medical doctor, used to joke that some of his psychiatrist friends were crazier than their patients. I'd say that Len is crazy like a fox. Confronted with the need to counter a rapidly aging body, most people would follow the herd and do what everybody does (jog, bike, swim, lift weights), but not Len Schwartz. Uniquely, he stepped back, surveyed and re-thought the fitness problem— and invented something new and wonderfully effective.

Knowing that his thoughts would be perceptive, enlightening and unconventional, I asked Len for his take on self challenge. I believe you'll agree, he did not disappoint.

"Two decades of 'active' interest in exercise have left me with a few notions that might be worth passing on. If one is interested in challenging oneself or perhaps instinctively a self challenging type, exercise may be both the best and worst of tactics! The good news is that almost anyone, in even the most dilapidated condition, can profit from 'appropriate' exercise. The bad news is that almost every exerciser, however resolute in the beginning, is fully capable of quitting the best program going!

"Part of it may be related to certain physiologic realities. The fact is that the poorer your level of fitness the greater your initial progress. And expectably, the better you get the more grudging the gains. Given those facts, I view lifelong exercisers as

218

unsung heros in our midst! They work the hardest, ofttimes despite the least in the way of tangible rewards!

"I began exercise better than 20 years ago as a 50-year-old runner. I quickly got to my 'physiologic sticking point.' Of course, I could interest myself in more scenic trails, ferreting out more optimal footwear, or watching the slow descent of my pulse rate. But running per se never promised much as far as my whole body strength, or other offbeat parameters like upper body aerobics.

"In my case a very sore set of hamstrings came to my rescue. It amounted to adding a handweight 'assist' to conventional exercise like jog or walk. By 'pumping' gradually increasing weights during my walks I killed a few ergometric birds with one stone: I could continue to challenge my heart with respectable continuous workloads despite my lame leg, preserve, perhaps enhance the musculature I had begun to develop as an adolescent, and as things turned out, begin a couple of decades of experiment with a novel kind of whole body exercise that captured gradual gains in endurance, strength and flexibility during every workout.

"My initial foray into modest weight training at 16 sort of petered out during college and medical school. I did remain faithful to a ritual of a few standard push-ups on days when I remembered! But that was it until somewhere in my late 40s. I rigged up one of those door jamb chinning bars in my office and added a few daily chins to my push-up ritual. Between 20 and 50, my exercise could have been characterized as spotty, sporadic, brief strength sprints; nothing that lasted longer than a minute!

"My personal experiment in physical challenge a la exercise must have happened when my earlier rather puny excursion into strength training collided with the new popularity of aerobics, courtesy Dr. Ken Cooper. That 'fortunate' hamstring injury actually shaped my thinking: I wanted to fashion for myself and for anyone else who was interested, a technique that would include whole-body strength, 'cardio' and flexibility.

"I wanted to fashion for myself and for anyone else who was interested, a technique that would include whole-body strength, 'cardio' and flexibility."

"That ambition led to bunches of (in hindsight) wonderful mini-experiments that soon turned into serious laboratory research and the writing of the first text on Heavyhands, the concept, and later the development of the glovelike dumbbell hardware called Heavyhands. I have to say that without that early strength implant in my soul and spirit, the subsequent amalgam I called Heavyhands could never have occurred.

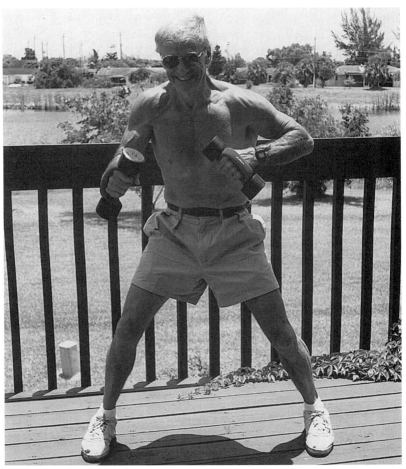

Now 74, Dr. Schwartz says he hasn't lost "a single gram of skeletal muscle." *Photo courtesy Len Schwartz, M.D.*

"So the business of self challenge in terms of physical improvement got linked solidly to science for me; found me moving happily into the world's exercise literature, occasionally submitting myself as a laboratory 'subject' to learn precisely where my weird exercise was taking me.

"Now at 74, I kind of consider myself something of an experimental animal. I work out anywhere from an hour to two hours every day. These workouts are highly varied, partly to preserve my enthusiasm, partly to gather new skills, partly to find out what this does for my 'numbers,' which continue to interest me in connection with my writing.

"My training, consisting of whole body routines that fuse strength with aerobics, is about as far removed from the bodybuilder's 'splits' as one can imagine. I avoid 'concentration curls' like the plague but enjoy watching others do them! For better or for worse, my ploy has to do with integrating rather than isolating muscles. And music is a constant vehicle for my workouts.

"Exercise has done 'right' by me! I hang on to my 40 resting pulse rate, skin fold fat of around 5% or less, a lowish blood pressure that had always been high. Also, I treasure a continued enjoyment of sports, i.e., serious rowing, touch football or baseball or tennis workouts with my adolescent grandchildren.

> "It has become clear that becoming a consistent self-challenger is important if not crucial in human development."

"What frankly excites me more are a few performances that continue to inch upward despite my age. And I have not—whatever the lexicons teach—lost a single gram of skeletal muscle.

"My late career change, a rather abrupt shift from my psychiatric practice to full time dealing with the theory and practice of exercise, has taught me a few things. For one, it has become clear that becoming a consistent self-challenger is important if not crucial in human development. For some of us developmental progress is easier to manage and measure in the bodily arena where change can be monitored confidently. I believe that body development may in time become a paradigm for all sorts of development.

"There is a lot of literature and clinical experience suggesting powerfully that good bodies make their hosts smarter in some ways! Wise physique management can't be far away from other forms of wisdom, and all the brain power in the world seems somehow diluted when the host's body has been chronically ignored. I continue to believe that lifelong exercise is the premier wellness strategy, better than all the others because it tends to mobilize them, too!"

Thanks, Len. I don't believe we could find a more insightful and encouraging way to end a book on self challenge.

CHALLENGE YOURSELF!

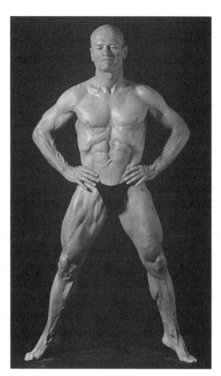

The photos on this page and those on the next two pages, *all by Pat Berrett*, are from my latest photo session, shortly after I turned 60. They show what you can accomplish if you CHALLENGE YOURSELF.

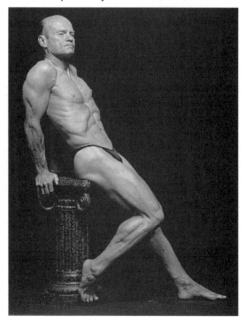

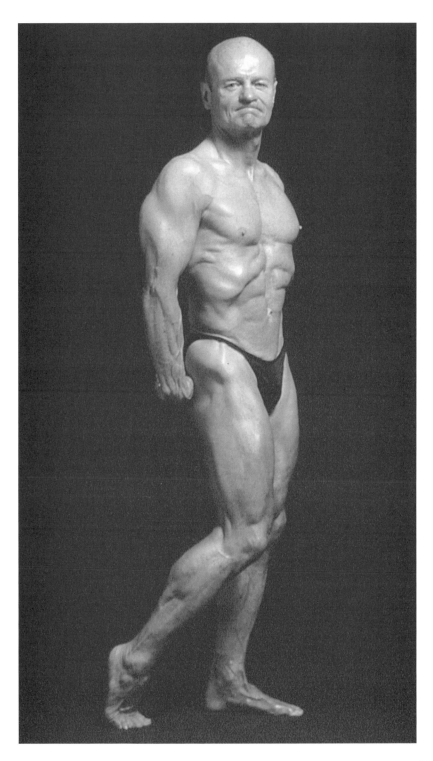

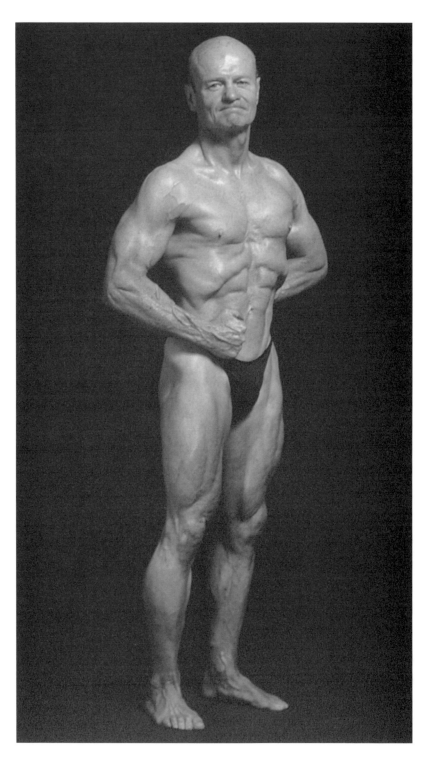

Other books by Clarence Bass

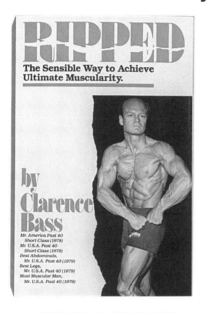

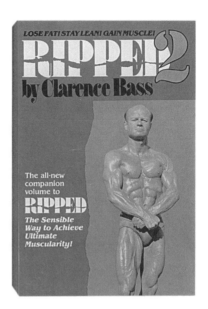

THE RIPPED SERIES

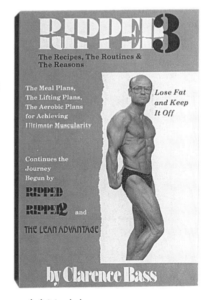

Clarence Bass' quest for lifelong leanness begins with the *Ripped* series. Your journey should begin there as well.

In **Ripped**, Clarence explains, step-by-step, how he reduced his body fat to 2.4% and won his class in the Past-40 Mr. America contest. This is the basic diet book for bodybuilders and fitness-minded individuals.

Ripped 2 explains staying lean, aerobics, building muscle, peaking and bodybuilding psychology. Many say it's the best book ever written on weight training.

Ripped 3 contains detailed comments on 22 meal plans that will make and keep you lean. Plus, it's the breakthrough book on periodization training for bodybuilders.

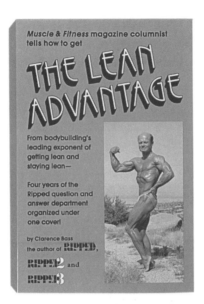
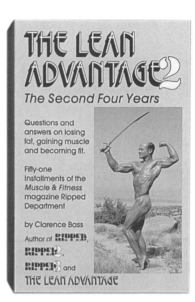
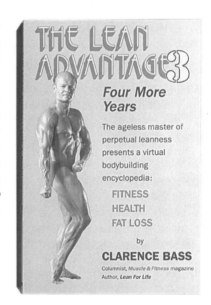

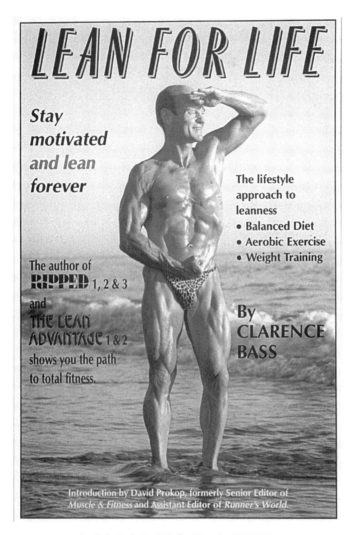

LEAN FOR LIFE

The fitness trend is toward balanced training—strength and endurance. Clarence Bass leads the way with *LEAN FOR LIFE.* He explains, day-by-day, how to combine weights and aerobics to achieve total fitness. What's more, he shows how to stay motivated — and lean — forever. He presents a lifestyle approach that *will make you lean for life!*

Don't miss a single step on the road to permanent leanness. Read all of Clarence Bass' books.

Turn page for more information and where to order.

Clarence Bass' RIPPED™ Enterprises

Is now on the web!
Please visit us at http://www.cbass.com

You'll find not only information about our books and other products, but also more about Clarence Bass' background and training career, his diet and training philosophy in brief, frequently asked questions, late news — and new articles by Clarence Bass (a new article at the beginning of each month). We are your source for bodybuilding, fitness, health, motivation, diet and fat loss information

Also available from
**Clarence Bass' RIPPED
Enterprises**

❖ Posing Trunks

❖ Women's Posing Suits

❖ Audio Tapes

❖ Color Photos

❖ Food Supplements

❖ Selected Books

❖ Personal Consultations

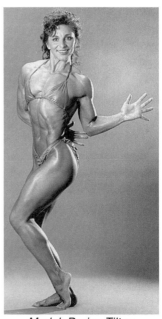

Model: Dorine Tilton

Clarence Bass' RIPPED Enterprises
528 Chama NE
Albuquerque, NM 87108 USA
Phone: 505-266-5858 / Fax: 505-266-9123

E-mail: cncbass@aol.com
Web site: http://www.cbass.com